YOUR BODY IN MIND

YOUR BODY
IN MIND

by

Marilyn Brannin

The Key to Health and Happiness
through Body Sense Therapy

SOUVENIR PRESS

First published 1982 by Souvenir Press Ltd,
43 Great Russell Street, London WC1B 3PA
and simultaneously in Canada

ISBN 0 285 62498 9

Photoset and printed in Great Britain by
Photobooks (Bristol) Ltd,
28 Midland Road, St Philips, Bristol

CONTENTS

INTRODUCTION

How to use this book

I have written this book to tell you how your body can give you perfect health – provided you give it the chance to do so. Body Sense Therapy puts you in touch with yourself, makes you aware of your true physical and psychological needs and allows you to tap the healing powers that lie within each and every one of us. It is the royal road to healthy living that anybody who wishes may travel with ease. Before describing the techniques involved I want to start by explaining the layout of the book. Simply, it has been split into six parts, each of which explores some specific aspect of wellbeing and outlines the procedures to follow in straightforward, step-by-step instructions supported by illustrations.

In Part One I am going to show you how you may either greatly alleviate or successfully eliminate a whole host of everyday pains. You will discover how to ease away headaches, neck stiffness, backpains and the uncomfortable symptoms associated with colds or hayfever. I am starting with a discussion of pain relief since it is almost impossible to feel good about your body when one area of it is giving you a bad time.

In Part Two you will learn how various massage techniques can be used to release your body's natural powers of healing. This section will provide you with the insights needed for the remaining four parts of the book, each of which deals with a key aspect of mental or physical health.

Part Three includes advice on investigating the way in which your body performs everyday activities so as to enable you to detect impending problems at the earliest possible moment. I will then reveal how, using Body Sense methods, any difficulties you do discover can be eliminated long before they reach the point of making your life miserable. My clients tell me that, by setting aside a few minutes each day for these easy exercises, they are able to escape most of the aches and pains which afflict their friends.

Part Four looks at ways of reducing the harmful effects of stress. I will explain how damaging muscle tensions, which excessive anxiety produces, can undermine your fitness. I will also describe a variety of procedures which will allow you to cope confidently with all kinds of stressful situations and emerge unscathed from encounters that might, previously, have left you a nervous wreck.

In Part Five I want to talk about your appearance and show you how Body Sense techniques can not only make you feel good but look good as well. This is important because the way you look reflects the health of your system. A poor complexion and posture speak volumes about the body responsible for them. People who appear below their best usually feel and function poorly as well.

I am sure you are familiar with the morale-boosting effect of an improved appearance and this is the chief reason why it is important to feel good about the way you look. How you regard your body exerts a powerful influence on the way you treat your body. If you are depressed about your appearance you are unlikely to heed your innermost needs. You will want to shut out messages about yourself from your mind. As a result, distress signals must become very powerful before any attention is paid to them – by which time the damage to health will be much harder to put right.

I want you to love your own body. Not in a narcissistic way but sensibly and realistically. I want you to love yourself because only if you feel *that* good about your body will you truly want it to function efficiently and healthily. It is almost impossible to experience strong, positive emotions about somebody we despise and that applies to self-love as well. So start looking your best and you are more likely to begin treating yourself for the best.

In Part Six I will show you how Body Sense techniques can be used to create *whole body health*. You will learn a series of massage and movement techniques which have proved their health-enhancing value, in some cases for more than a thousand years. All are easy to perform, pleasantly relaxing and absolutely non-strenuous. If however you are receiving medical treatment for any reason, check with your doctor that it will be safe to undertake these exercises. Such a precaution is also sensible if you have high blood pressure, are overweight or have any history of heart disease.

Looking through the book you may, initially, feel a little daunted by all the exercises I describe. Perhaps you wonder if all have to be mastered and how long it would take to do them. Well, this book is intended to be your companion in healthy living for a long time to come, which is why I have put so much into it. But you should take out *only* those exercises which are necessary to achieve and then sustain a sense of wellbeing. For instance, if you are fortunate enough to be completely free of discomforting pains at this moment then skip Part One and go directly to Part Two. If you are unlucky enough to suffer from some discomfort later, then you can refer to the appropriate technique in Part One and use it to alleviate the problem.

I suggest you read through all the parts quite rapidly and in a relaxed manner to get an overall idea of the tremendous benefits which can be derived from Body Sense Therapy. Then use this knowledge, together with the index, to plan an appropriate course of exercises that occupy the amount of time each day you could devote to your health care. To make this planning easier most of the exercises have been timed. Use this programme as long as you feel the need for it but do not be afraid to change the exercises to match changing bodily requirements. In this way you develop a timetable which exactly matches your highly individual bodily needs.

Now I hope you are ready and eager to make a start.

Welcome to the world of Body Sense Therapy and a new life of health and beauty.

Body Sense therapy – your natural way to perfect health

Perfect health is the most natural thing in the world – and the most elusive. Many people spend their lives searching unsuccessfully for mental and physical fitness. They range far and wide in their quest for some pill, potion or remedy that will alleviate nagging discomforts, ease distressing anxieties and enable them to feel completely alive again. Sadly such efforts are a waste of time and energy. Perfect health is not hidden in any bottle or jar. It cannot be found on the pharmacist's shelves, in the doctor's consulting room or the club gymnasium. You cannot buy well-being, nor is there any need to do so. The irony of this hunt for health is that the eager searchers already possess the very thing they so desperately seek. The secret of absolute fitness is locked away inside each one of us. All we need to discover is the best way of liberating the natural powers of the human body.

I call the means by which these potent forces can be released and used Body Sense Therapy. During my years as a health and beauty specialist I have shown people from all walks of life how to use its simple, straightforward procedures. My clients, who include movie stars, international business executives, housewives and even doctors, have discovered that Body Sense therapy gives them the sensation of radiant well-being that makes life a pleasure to savour rather than an ordeal to be survived. Now I want to explain how the same procedures will quickly and easily work to relieve everyday pains, reduce stressful tensions, and help you live life to the full. By following the methods I describe, and setting aside just a few minutes each day to put them into practice, you too will be able to help yourself to health.

Let me start by asking you a question I sometimes put to my clients, occasionally with unexpected results: Are you living on intimate terms with a stranger? Do you share your life with a close companion you hardly know, seldom listen to and frequently abuse?

You can see why this query leads to some odd looks and surprising replies! But the truth is most people are in this position. They are barely on speaking terms with a lifetime partner whose innermost needs and true feelings remain forever a mystery to them. The stranger I am talking about is your own body! Before you protest that such a notion is nonsense and insist that you are responsive to your bodily requirements and sensitive to its needs, ask yourself this question: When was the last time you seriously paid attention to something your body wanted to tell you? My guess is that the most vivid recent memory is of a cry for help. A time when something went wrong and the normally unobtrusive system started to break down. Alarm signals rang noisily in your brain. An ailment or infection made life miserable. For a while you listened to and acted on what your body was saying. Then the ache or pain vanished, the discomfort disappeared, sickness subsided and you began to take yourself for granted all over again.

Most people mistreat themselves in this way. They turn a deaf ear to signals from the body, reluctantly acknowledging these inner messages only when they have become too urgent and uncomfortable to be ignored any longer. As a result they spend a lot of time neither looking nor feeling truly healthy. They may suffer from frequent headaches, poor digestion, an unending succession of colds; they get easily tired, live on their nerves and age unnecessarily early.

If this sounds rather familiar do not be too depressed. None of these conditions is unavoidable. Life does not have to be like that. You *can* unlock your natural powers of good health by working with your body rather than against it; by learning how to use it in the way nature intended and discovering how to tune in to the signals from your inner self.

I have called this approach to well-being *Body Sense* because the term expresses the key to the two major techniques which are brought together in the therapy. The first refers to that interior *sense*, or wisdom, which is nature's gift to each of us. Your body is wise. It was built to work effortlessly and efficiently. It knows when something has gone wrong and how best to put matters right. It tries to communicate these warnings but usually fails to get through because you are either unable or unwilling to pay attention to its murmured messages. This brings me to the second meaning of Body Sense, that of *sensation*, the constant flow of messages from within that can be used to keep in touch with your innermost needs.

By mastering the techniques of Body Sense Therapy you help yourself to health in three vitally important ways:

*You will learn how to detect the faint, early signals when something goes wrong so that potential health hazards can be eliminated, often long before they are able to exert any harmful effects.

*You will discover how to tap your body's inbuilt health giving forces, so as to ease away everyday aches and pains without turning to drugs. By using your powers of self-healing it becomes possible to relieve symptoms caused by headaches, stiff muscles, cramps, digestive problems and colds, among many other familiar discomforts. While not serious in themselves, such symptoms can easily make you vulnerable to more serious health problems.

*You will develop a sensitivity to your body which ensures you work together in harmony, responsive to its needs and able to carry out everyday activities with an ease that enhances mental and physical fitness.

A healthy body is one working as nature intended, under the control of a brain tuned to its most subtle messages. Body Sense therapy will bring about this perfect union by giving you insight into the two vital systems on which wellbeing depends. The first consists of the muscle groups that make up more than half our total weight and the second is the network of sense organs that provide the mind with information about how well those muscles are working. This network of nerves makes up . . .

The sixth sense we never think about

Everybody is familiar with the five senses, of seeing, hearing, tasting, touching and smelling, that tell us what is happening in our surroundings. For knowledge of what is happening inside ourselves we rely on this sixth sense, a complex system of detectors, built into the muscles, which provide the brain with information about every aspect of bodily function. Scientists call it the *kinesthetic system* and it has been the subject of intense interest and study for more than a century.

A hundred years ago it was realised that the muscles work in response to commands from the brain which are transmitted via impulses in the nerves. But it is only more recently that studies have revealed muscles also communicate with the brain along these same pathways. Some of the delicate sensors in muscles and ligaments respond to every change in tension and stretch, while others send the brain information about the position of the limbs; still others keep a check on the amount of effort being used to perform everyday activities. If we try to do something which is physically too demanding and might cause harm – lifting too heavy a weight for example – these sensors send the brain a rapid order to stop. We can survive and even flourish if blind or deaf, and overcome the loss of the sensations of taste, touch or smell, but if we lost the sixth sense then life itself would become impossible.

Get back in touch with that sense of self

If you are absorbed in a thriller you will probably be unaware of your surroundings. At a crowded party you can easily focus your attention on just one conversation and ignore the babble all around.

In much the same way it is possible to concentrate on the information coming from your fingertips, your mouth – as when you are eating something delicious – or your nostrils. By directing the mind to a particular sensation in this way you shut out competing demands for attention from the other senses.

While this is the most natural thing to do, and indeed essential for our survival on many occasions, it works to the disadvantage of the sixth sense. Because we are so attentive to signals from the other five, its messages tend to be ignored. If we are to get in touch with our inner selves, and listen to those vital facts about the way our body is working, we must learn how to turn attention inwards rather than outwards. It is only by enhancing sensitivity and responsiveness to the sixth sense that we can start using our body efficiently.

How Sixth Sense Works

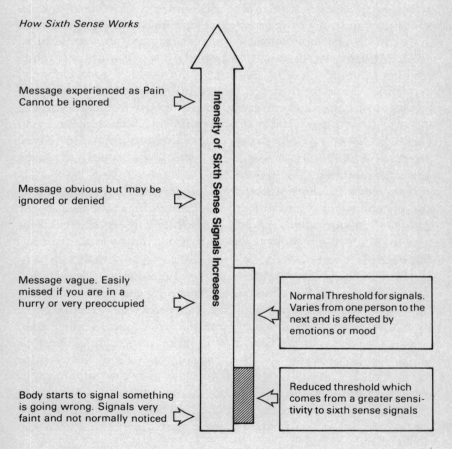

Message experienced as Pain
Cannot be ignored

Message obvious but may be
ignored or denied

Message vague. Easily
missed if you are in a
hurry or very preoccupied

Body starts to signal something
is going wrong. Signals very
faint and not normally noticed

Intensity of Sixth Sense Signals Increases

Normal Threshold for signals.
Varies from one person to the
next and is affected by
emotions or mood

Reduced threshold which
comes from a greater sensitivity to sixth sense signals

As you can see, the first faint signals of distress are very hard to detect and will normally be ignored. As the intensity of the sixth sense messages increases we are more likely to take notice of them, but our awareness will be influenced by emotional factors. Beyond a certain point, however, the signals are experienced as pain which usually increases until it simply cannot be ignored. Sensitivity training allows you to lower the threshold of awareness so that you detect the messages far earlier and are thus in a much stronger position to prevent the problem from developing further. In this way you can avoid much discomfort and distress while effectively safeguarding your health.

With practice it soon becomes possible to tune into the sixth sense at any convenient moment. You will find it as easy to focus your attention inwards as you do at the moment to concentrate on anything important in your external surroundings. Checks on the body can then be made whenever you have a spare moment: walking down a street, perhaps, or sitting behind a desk, in your car or while relaxing at home.

At first, however, you will probably find it easier to pick up messages with the inner ear if you 'turn down' the volume control of the other five senses. The best way to do this is to choose a quiet room with a bed or chair so that you can relax comfortably. Some people also like to draw the blinds. Take off your shoes and loosen any tight clothing.

Now sit or lie quite still and spend a few moments relaxing as completely as possible. To distract your mind from the cares of the day try to picture some tranquil scene. After a few moments I want you to begin to concentrate on your head and face. Start at the forehead. Is it tense or relaxed? Move to the eyes. Are they tired or strained? Now go to the mouth and jaw. Focus on your tongue and your teeth. Spend a few moments just thinking about each part of the head then go on to the body. Notice any sensations of discomfort or distress being communicated from that area. Localise such aches or pains as exactly as possible. Do not think, for example: I've got a stiff back. Pinpoint the source of the stiffness. Is it in the upper or lower back? If upper, does it include the neck and shoulders? If lower, are the hips and thighs also uncomfortable?

Work methodically around the body. There is no need to spend more than a few seconds on each part. If no discomfort is experienced you may then move quickly on. Pay special attention to the neck and shoulders as these are places where normally unnoticed tensions tend to develop and lead to headaches. Think about your fingers and hands, your wrists and elbows. Move from the chest and upper back to the abdomen and lower spinal region. Progress down the legs. Focus on your knees, shins, ankles and toes.

Even at the start it need take no more than a few minutes to perform a complete and thorough check. When you are experienced at tuning in to the sixth sense you will find it possible to focus instantly on these areas where distress signals are being emitted.

If you detect areas of discomfort, however trivial, make a mental note of them. At the end of the session I suggest you keep a more permanent record of the trouble spot by making notes about its condition and rate of recovery. Many people find it helpful to keep a "Body Sense notebook" in which they record their progress from month to month. This need not be done in great detail – just note down the most important details. By carrying out the Body Sense techniques described in this book you will be able to help eliminate difficulties in just a few sessions. You will be able to alleviate distress and prevent problems from getting worse by using the appropriate methods.

Using the sixth sense to check out allergies

Do some foods disagree with you? Is your body upset by certain kinds of drinks? By tobacco? Or when in close proximity to a particular substance? Very often we suffer from an allergic reaction without being aware of what causes the problem. Foods which we enjoy, but are actually harmful to our system, can be eaten regularly without ever being linked to the discomfort or distress they cause.

But your body always knows, and, if you are prepared to listen to the sixth sense in the right way, is able to warn you of the dangers. To demonstrate just how sensitive the sense really is and to show yet another way in which it can help safeguard health, I am going to describe a simple technique for detecting this type of allergic response.

To carry out the test you will need help from a friend. Stand with your arms outstretched, palms down, and have her push down diagonally sideways on your wrists. You should be able to resist this pressure fairly easily. Now introduce the substance you want to check. If it is food or drink place a little on the tongue. If it is something like tobacco then simply bring it close to the body. Your sixth sense will detect the danger and signal instantly by causing a loss of strength in the arm muscles. Instead of successfully pushing up against your friend's downward pressure, your arms will lose their resistance. The stronger the reaction the more powerful the response. I have seen a person allergic to tobacco, for example, whose arms lost their strength when a packet of cigarettes was placed on the upper arm. This is a very easy technique to carry out, and I have never known it to fail. Test a few of the foodstuffs which form a part of your regular diet and you may be surprised by what you discover. Interpret any loss of resistance in the arm muscles as a clear sixth sense warning to avoid that food in the future.

The sixth sense gives us essential knowledge about how our *muscles* are working. Although these are not usually parts of the body associated with good health, except perhaps by weightlifters or gymnasts, they actually hold the key to fitness for us all. Physical and mental wellbeing depend not on bulging biceps and calves like tree trunks, but on muscles which are capable of working at a peak efficiency. A healthy body is one in which the muscles are in perfect health themselves.

Why muscle health is so important

A major emphasis in Body Sense Therapy is the improvement of muscle function through techniques of massage and movement. Why do I stress its importance? An obvious answer might be because muscles make up such a large part of the body and we can only enjoy an active life through their carefully controlled use. But they do far more than just move us around. Each of the more than 150 muscles in the human body is a fantastic biological factory, transforming the raw materials of glucose and oxygen into mechanical work, regulating bodily heat, storing energy supplies and controlling the chemistry of the body in a very precise manner. Dr P. M. Daniel of the Royal College of Surgeons in London, one of the world's leading authorities on muscle, has remarked that these tasks, although little understood and seldom appreciated, are just as crucial to life as the part muscles play in supporting the skeleton and moving the body about. Consider, for instance, an activity as crucial to survival as the circulation of the blood. We all know that this depends on the pumping action of the heart. Much less well known is the fact that other muscles, especially those in the legs, are also involved in circulating blood round the body. So essential is the contribution of this 'muscle pump' that, should it be turned off, the heart alone is often unable to cope with the demands made upon it. Soldiers standing to attention on parade faint because the muscles in the legs are unable to help the heart pump blood against the force of gravity. Too little reaches the brain which is starved of oxygen and energy foods. The body responds by fainting. This brings the head below the level of the feet, eliminates the problem of gravity and restores the blood flow to the head.

So strong, healthy leg muscles not only allow you to walk further or run faster, they also keep the heart in good condition. This leads to efficient circulation of the blood enabling plenty of oxygen and glucose to reach all parts of the body. As a result you are able to think quickly and clearly; naturally-produced poisons are effectively removed from the cells and every part of the body receives the nutrients on which their health depends. Maintaining the right level of blood pressure also means that organs like the kidneys and liver can work properly.

To bring your muscles into good condition there is no need to go jogging for miles, lift weights or engage in strenuous exercise. I am going to tell you how such health can be achieved and sustained by doing little more in the way of daily activities than you do already.

The no-effort way to muscle health

Professor Allen Ryan of the University of Wisconsin, one of America's leading physical education specialists, has shown in experiments that when muscles are at rest they immediately begin to lose their tone: that is, the essential tension they must maintain in order to function at maximum efficiency. Professor Ryan has also found that to maintain a healthy level of tone, the muscles must produce movements involving continuous tension. This is not the way most people use them. On the contrary, the average person carries out activities in a series of abrupt rapid, and jerky movements with tiny rest pauses between them. These are so slight that we are normally unaware of them in ourselves or others. To the unaided eye it may seem that each action is a continuous flow of movement. But it is not and this shows up in the damaging effects on the muscles as they alternate between a state of tension and relaxation.

An equally serious problem, which arises from the demands of modern life, is that large groups of muscles may remain unused for long periods as their owner sits behind a desk or at the wheel of a car, or stands at a kitchen sink or factory bench. Professor Ryan found that remaining motionless in this way is actually *more* exhausting for the muscles than moving around. They have a natural need to work regularly in order to remain healthy. When obliged to work irregularly or move incorrectly deterioration of performance is inevitable.

So here are two ways you can help your muscles – and hence your whole body – stay in shape without expending any additional effort.

If you have to sit or stand still for long periods then set aside a few moments for exercising every muscle group. This can be done without any special equipment and there is no need even to raise a sweat. Just work through the body in a methodical fashion. I suggest you begin with your fingers and toes. Wriggle them. Now exercise wrists and ankles. Circle them a few times. Flex and stretch them. Straighten your arms, bend and straighten them again. Move up to the shoulders. Shrug them using circular movements. Squeeze your buttocks together and flatten your stomach. Walk around for a few moments stretching your spine as you do so. This need take no more than a few seconds yet if carried out three or four times each day these exercises alone could add years to your life and prove of tremendous benefit to your general health.

But exercise, while important, is not the only consideration. How you carry out these, and any other, activities is equally significant. Bear in mind the harm done to muscle tone by movements which are abrupt. Watch how other people perform many everyday tasks – and avoid the same mistakes. Instead of copying their general effortful and inefficient actions, imitate a cat. Observe how these beautiful creatures seem almost to flow across the ground like trickles of quicksilver. Now compare the way you move to their relaxed grace and, while performing your muscle toning movements each day, be certain you do so in an equally effortless and elegant way. Avoid unnecessary tensions by allowing those parts of the body not being used at that moment to remain relaxed. Once this simple skill has been mastered you should have no problem at all in carrying it through to everyday activities.

As your powers of sixth sense develop, harmful and unnatural movements become less likely because you will be much more aware of the messages of protest coming from the mistreated muscles. Your posture will then improve and you will move with a more natural grace and agility.

So let's get started. Your way to perfect health begins on the very next page.

PART ONE

The Body Sense way

Important note: Remember that pain is a warning. These techniques will help remove distressing symptoms but, in many cases, they are not going to remove the underlying cause. If discomfort persists or recurs frequently the *only* safe and sensible course is to go and talk things over with your doctor. Prompt attention to minor difficulties can frequently prevent them from becoming more serious.

You cannot feel good about life if your body feels badly about it! Even relatively minor aches and pains, when persistent, lead to a decrease in energy, an inability to concentrate, and a jaded outlook on life. So we must begin by alleviating such discomfort as much as possible. Looking through the case notes of my clients, I find that a number of different problems seem to crop up again and again. So in this part of the book I am going to describe the Body Sense approach to relieving these familiar symptoms:
Muscle spasms;

headaches;

strained and tired eyes;

toothache;

facial pains;

asthma;

cold and hayfever symptoms;

sinus pains;

neck stiffness;

shoulder pains;

stomach pains (including travel sickness);

constipation;

shin splints;

hand, arm and elbow pains (including tennis and golfer's elbow);

back pain;

sciatica pain;
knee pain.

In the past you may have tried to cope with ailments of this kind in one of two ways. Perhaps you attempted the stoical 'forget all about it and keep on going' approach. You did your best to ignore the pains and carried on as well as you could until the problem disappeared. Busy people with responsibilities cannot retire from daily life just because they feel slightly unwell, so you may not have had much choice in the matter. It is also not unlikely that you tried to help yourself over the bad times through the use of various patent painkillers and symptom relievers such as aspirins and cold cures, embrocations and liniments, indigestion tablets and antisickness pills. These at least masked the pain and discomfort even if they did nothing to treat the root cause of the problems.

Body Sense Therapy offers a more natural and comfortable way of dealing with these everyday aches and pains. The techniques I am going to describe allow you to tap the natural healing power within your body, which is then able to cure itself, sometimes in a matter of minutes. But before carrying out any of these self-help methods please bear in mind four important points:

One:

There is little purpose in relieving a particular pain if your present way of living is such that it causes the same problem to occur again and again. A tension headache, for instance, can be quickly alleviated using the procedures I describe. But if you are under a great deal of stress it is bound to return. So make certain you use these, essentially first-aid, remedies in conjunction with the techniques described later in the book, which are designed to bring about permanent improvements in mental and physical health.

Two:

The treatments I outline often consist of a series of individual techniques designed to tackle a specific ache or pain. To obtain full benefit you must complete the sequence of massages described.

Three:

If the pains persist, or if any of the techniques causes you discomfort, then make an appointment to *see your doctor*.

Remember that pain is a warning. It may be a signal of some relatively trivial and transitory breakdown in bodily efficiency. But it is also possible that the message is alerting you to a problem serious enough to require professional help to put it right. Never take chances with your health.

Four:

Finally a word of warning about massaging the stomach if you are pregnant, or have recently undergone abdominal surgery. Once again the best advice is to consult your doctor if in any doubt.

The treatments

For the sake of convenience I am going to approach pain relief by starting with the head and working down the body. First though I shall begin by describing a useful general massage procedure whose purpose is to release muscle spasm, a common condition which accompanies many types of aches and pains.

Releasing muscle spasm

Muscle tissue is usually soft and pliable, but following injury, such as a knock or a twist, a small, hard, painful knot can appear. This may be the size of a *golf-ball*. It is called a *spasm* and you will need to restore the muscle to its normal feel and appearance in order to ease away the discomfort this condition causes.

You can locate the spasm quite easily by running your fingers down the muscle. To release it, stroke the area gently but firmly in the direction of the heart. Continue the stroking for 15 seconds. Should this fail to reduce the spasm, press your thumb firmly into the widest part of the muscle for 30 seconds. If it still persists, press the knot directly, again using your thumb, for a further 30 seconds. Complete the massage with 15 seconds of gentle stroking over the whole area. This should release the spasm and alleviate the pain.

Now let us begin our quest for fast pain relief by starting at the top.

Headaches

These are probably the most common health problem I am asked to deal with. Medical experts say that more than three quarters of the world's population are prone to headaches, and I believe them! Time after time clients plead: 'Before you do anything else, please help me get rid of this terrible head pain.'

Headaches quickly reduce your ability to concentrate, making it impossible to enjoy life. Your nerves feel as if they have been fed through a shredder. They are unpleasant for you and often equally difficult for your family and friends.

Interestingly, the brain – although it makes us aware of pain – cannot feel any pain itself. The ache is caused either by inflamation of the delicate membranes which surround it, poisons in the blood which bathes it, pressure in the delicate bones of the sinus, or by tension in the muscles of the neck and scalp.

The three most common types of headache, which can all be effectively alleviated using Body Sense Therapy, are due to tensions and pressures in the head and neck.

Tension headaches

These pains are caused by unnecessary tautness of the neck and face muscles. This may be due to emotional stress – the struggle to conceal our true feelings places the facial muscles under consider-able tension – or long periods of concentration during which the face is set in a fixed mask. As you grow more accustomed to sixth sense signals, you will become increasingly aware of these needless tensions and your automatic response to the first faint murmurings of muscular distress will be to relax. This should greatly reduce the number and severity of tension head pains.

Eye strain headaches

Here again the villain is needless tension. It may be that you are tired and having to strain the delicate eye muscles in order to focus properly; or there could be a defect in your vision of which you are unaware. It makes sense to have your eyes checked regularly by an optician, especially as you get older. Head pains can also arise if you expose the eyes to ultra-violet light, for example by looking directly at the sun, for only a few seconds. This kind of headache can last up to 48 hours.

As you grow more sensitive to sixth sense messages, tiny distress signals from the eye muscles will be easier to detect and you will be able to eliminate this type of problem by removing the tensions responsible.

Infection headaches

The cause of the problem here is pressure in the sinuses and the membranes lining the nose. This is the sort of headache you get when suffering from colds or hayfever, sinusitis and any infection which causes the build up of mucus. Such pains may be felt behind the eyes or around the front of the scalp and forehead.

Relieving headaches

Before using pressure point massage for the headache problems described above, here is a general exercise with which you should start your treatment and which is designed to ease away tension in the face and neck muscles. In some instances you may find that nothing further is necessary as the pain will have completely vanished during the course of relaxation. When you have trained in Body Sense awareness for a few weeks, you will be able to detect tension headaches at such an early stage that relaxation alone should be sufficient to prevent any pain developing. The technique can be carried out anywhere and at any time but it works best when your whole body is relaxing in a hot bath.

Step one: Look directly ahead and raise your eyebrows as hard as you can, as though enquiring. Frown so as to tense the muscles in your forehead. Hold this tension for a slow count of five.

Step Two: Relax your forehead, scalp and facial muscles completely by looking down and lightly closing your eyes. Create a mental picture of warm water flowing soothingly down your forehead. Try to imagine this as vividly as possible and think how comforting it would feel.

Step Three: Now, keeping your face and scalp muscles as relaxed as you can, tense the neck muscles by turning down the corners of your mouth in a grimace. If this is done correctly it will make the cords at each side of the neck stand out noticeably. Once again hold the tension for a slow count of five before suddenly relaxing the muscles.

Then create the image of warm water lapping gently around your chin. If you are carrying out this technique in a bath you can, of course, immerse yourself to experience the real thing. Even so, you should still develop your ability to conjure up a powerful mental image so that you can use the sensation of warm water any time you want to relax the face and neck muscles.

Continue to relax as completely as possible for a few moments. Try listening to the sixth sense signals from your head, face and neck in order to detect any remaining traces of tension. By the end of this session your headache should have been eased considerably, if not entirely disappeared. If traces of pain persist continue the treatment with a short set of exercises designed to banish tension in the neck muscles:

One:

Sit on the floor with your back straight, one leg bent and the other stretched out in front of you. Clasp your arms around your bent knee bringing it close to your body and drop your head forward. (You should feel the muscles stretch right up the back of the neck.) Hold this position for about 12 seconds.

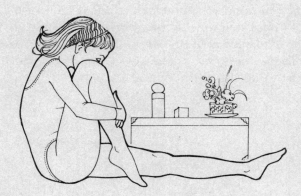

Fig. 1

Two:

Stretch the bent leg, clasp your hands behind your back and draw in your shoulders as far as you can while letting your head tilt backwards. Hold this position for 12 seconds.

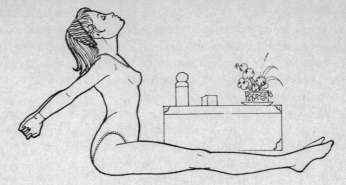

Fig. 2

Three:

Now relax completely and gently roll your head around, first in a clockwise and then in an anticlockwise direction.

If the headache is still present the next area of tension we must deal with is that around the scalp muscles. You can ease problems here by using a technique perfected in China to enhance the circulation of blood through the scalp and relax the whole area around the top of the head. Proceed as follows:

One:

Place your hands on either side of the head. Continue to breathe normally but listen to your breathing. Press firmly with both palms together, and *each time you inhale* lift the scalp on each side of the head. Every time *you exhale move hands and scalp downwards*. Continue to do this for about 30 seconds.

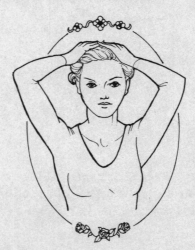

Fig. 3

Two:

Move the hands so that they press against the forehead and back of the head and carry out the same lift and drop movements as you breathe in and out for a further 30 seconds. Finish by massaging your toes and fingers until they are warm.

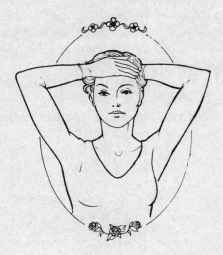

Fig. 4

If there are any remaining traces of the tension headache, carry out the following pressure point massage.

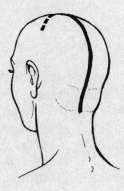

Fig. 5

You should begin by applying moderate pressure along the imaginary line (shown in Figure 5) which runs back along the middle of the scalp to the base of the skull. Starting at the hairline, press steadily with the four fingers of each hand on this line. At some points along the line you will notice a specially tender spot. This is the correct place to apply firm but gentle pressure for *two minutes*. Move your fingers back along the line, probing for the correct pressure points and pressing for two minutes on each one found.

On reaching the base of the skull use the thumb of each hand to probe the two bony protrusions there. If you detect a tender spot apply pressure for two minutes as before.

Next, explore for pressure points along two imaginary lines on each shoulder. It is best to tackle them one shoulder at a time since applying sufficient pressure with both hands is difficult. Once again probe for especially sensitive spots and then press them for two

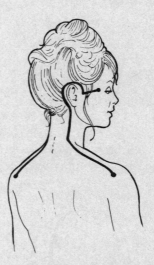

Fig. 6

minutes. As this is a part of the body where considerable tension can occur it is likely you will discover quite a number of sore points.

When you have completed this treatment, which need take no more than fifteen minutes, most types of headaches caused by tension in the neck, shoulders or scalp should have been much improved or completely relieved. Work through the list of treatments diligently and do not become discouraged if the pain persists right up to the last set of pressure point massages. It *will* be alleviated if the underlying cause is excessive tension in the major muscle groups I have described. (Fig. 6.)

There is, however, one further source of tension headaches that will require the help of your dentist to put right. This is a pain caused by excessive strain to the muscles and ligaments joining the upper and lower jaws which can be caused by a faulty alignment between the two. New York dentists Dr Harold Gelb and Dr Jeffrey Tarte have devised a simple test to allow this problem to be self-diagnosed.

All you have to do is place your little fingers in each ear and close your mouth. Now open and close it again. If the lower jaw is out of alignment you will hear a clicking noise. Should the diagnosis be positive, and you suffer from frequent headaches, this could be the cause of your problem. With the help of a dentist, the jaws can be realigned and muscle tension thereby relieved.

Tension headaches due to eye strain

If eye strain is the cause of your headaches it should be quite obvious because the pain will occur following any period of concentration. You can ease away the pain by using this simple technique developed by the yogis. *If you wear contact lenses it is essential to remove them before starting the treatment.*

One:

Rub your hands briskly together for about 30 seconds and then shake vigorously so as to warm them. Now place your palms over your closed eyes with the fingertips just touching the hairline as shown in Figure 7. Rest them there for 15 seconds.

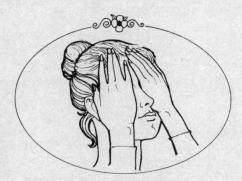

Fig. 7

Two:

Move your hands down so that the fingertips are just underneath the eyebrows. Push gently upwards right along the arch of the eyebrow. Gently and slowly stroke the lids outwards, towards the temples, using the fingertips. Repeat the stroking movement ten times. Then, keeping your eyes closed, relax your face for a few moments. If the pain persists repeat the massage a number of times.

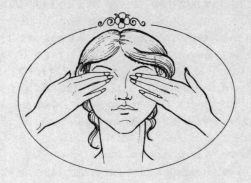

Fig. 8

Three:

Now, using the middle or index finger of both hands together, apply 5 seconds of gentle pressure to the hollows in the temples, which are located about half-an-inch from the corner of each eye. Next, place the fingers beneath each eye and make a circular stroking movement, following the directions of the arrows in Figure 8. Continue the circling until you reach the inner corners of the eyes. It is important to avoid stretching the skin, which is very delicate in this area. A helpful safeguard is to apply a small amount of face cream to your fingertips before starting.

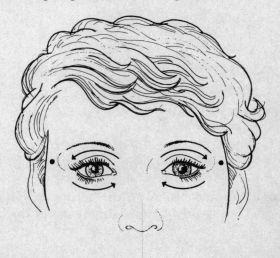

Fig. 9

At the end of this treatment the strained eye muscles will have been soothed back to health and your headache should have vanished. Remember, when carrying out your sixth sense training session, to focus on all the muscles in the head and face. These are so often placed under needless strain that tension pains are almost inevitable. This unnecessary stress also ages you prematurely by leading to a wrinkling and sagging of the skin.

Colds and hayfever

Here, I am going to describe a series of techniques which will help you to alleviate not only head pains but many of the other distressing symptoms caused by these problems. You should also find them helpful in the relief of sinus and asthma conditions.

Figure 10 shows four extremely important pressure points on the face which are directly in line with the pupils. They are to be found about one inch above the eyebrow; at the lower edge of the eyebrow; on the lower edge of the eye-socket; and directly under the lowest point of the cheekbone.

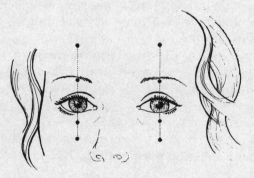

Fig. 10

Using the forefingers of both hands together apply moderate pressure to each of these points in turn for 2 minutes. Remember, when locating them, to seek out the specially tender spots in this area and to look for the little indentation beneath the skin which serve as your second signpost to specific pressure points. Next apply gentle pressure down each side of the nose from top to bottom for a total time of three minutes. This will help clear the nasal congestion.

Following the pressure point treatment with a very slow, deep friction massage, using both hands, down each side of the breast-

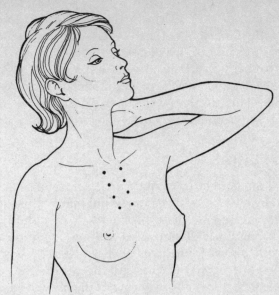

Fig. 11

bone. You should take plenty of time with this part of the treatment and it is best to do it twice. Check that you understand exactly what is involved with deep friction massage by reading my instructions on page 65 before starting.

After the massage to the breastbone move on to your ribs. Using the tips of the first three fingers, locate the grooves between your first, second and third ribs at the point where they join the breastbone.

Pressing fairly firmly, stroke outwards with both hands keeping your fingers in the grooves. The massage should be carried out slowly, so that it takes between 15 and 20 seconds, repeated several times.

The next part of the treatment consists of raising your hands above your head and panting rapidly like a dog on a hot day. This is a remarkably effective method of clearing upper respiratory congestion. Continue to pant for around 30 seconds.

At least twice a day, while you remain blocked up, practice what is called abdominal breathing. Take a couple of minutes to inhale and exhale in a way which is wonderfully effective in clearing away the congestion brought about by colds, 'flu or any type of respiratory infection. Do this as follows: Breath in by gently expanding your

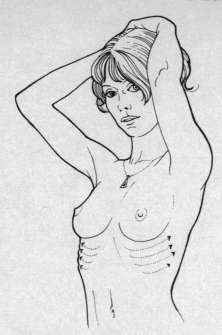

Fig. 12

abdomen while keeping the chest immobile. You will find this quite easy with only a little practice. Place your fingertips about two inches below your naval and start to inhale. If you are carrying out abdominal breathing correctly you will feel the abdomen expanding each time you take a breath. Develop this form or breathing as a regular part of your Body Sense programme. It helps expand the chest and releases muscle tensions. Most people who breathe poorly have rounded shoulders and overly tight chests.

By easing congestion in the sinuses you should go a long way to getting rid of tension headaches. But since sinus pains are often associated not only with headache but produce an aching dis-comfort around the whole area of the face, you should take steps to ease these facial pains as well.

Five points to prevention of facial pain

The illustration shows the location of five key points for the relief of facial pain. The numbers correspond with the technique below. Identify the precise spot on your own body by seeking out small indentations in the skin and/or specially tender places. Apply moderate pressure, using both index fingers at the same time, for a total of 2 minutes at each point.

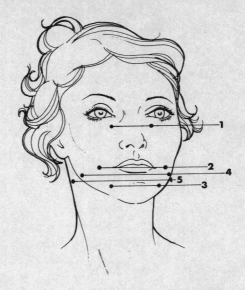

Fig. 13

One:
  Start here. The points are located either side of the nose a short distance down from the corners of the eyes.

Two:
  After two minutes, move to points located on the cheeks level with the edges of the mouth.

Three:
  Next move the fingers slightly forward and down to points along the curve of the chin.

Four:
  Now locate the pressure points just above the angle of the jaw.

Five:
  Finally identify the places which are on the neck about three finger widths from the ear lobes.
  Pressure in the sinuses is not the only possible cause of facial

pains. There could also be an underlying emotional difficulty as work by Dr. Stanley Lesse of Columbia University, New York, has shown. He found that people who experience frequent facial pains are often suffering from depression, without ever being aware of the fact. This psychological problem produces the physical discomfort which can only be treated effectively by tackling the depression itself. If persistent facial pains are a health problem you may find it helpful to make use of the techniques I shall describe in Part Five when I deal with stress.

Facial pains can, of course, also be due to toothache, the next sign of discomfort I am going to talk about.

Relieving toothache

As a first step you should phone your dentist and fix an appointment, but it makes sense to ease the discomfort as much as possible while waiting for treatment. Pressure point massage is a quick, effective method for bringing about such relief without the use of pain killers. One of the best techniques for alleviating dental pain acts on a major facial nerve (the trigeminal) by shutting off its signals. You perform the massage as follows:

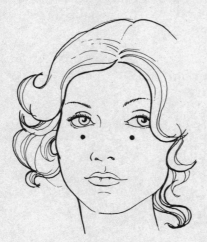

Fig. 14

Use this technique when the pain is in the *upper jaw*. Apply finger pressure to the points shown in Figure 14. These are located about half-an-inch from your nose and the same distance below your eyes. Keep up the pressure for two minutes having identified the most tender spot to press. You should feel the pain gradually ease away.

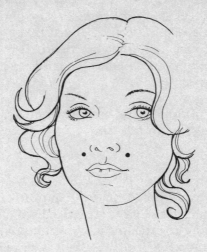

Fig. 15

When the pain is in the *lower jaw* apply pressure to the points located about half-an-inch from each nostril on a diagonal line from the nose. Probe gently around this area until your fingers feel the gum ridge. Two minutes of steady pressure should be maintained on points just above this ridge.

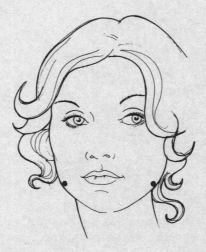

Fig. 16

After carrying out whichever of the above techniques is appropriate complete the treatment with pressure point massage designed to relieve pain in both jaws.

Find on the lower jaw, the two pressure points whose general position is shown in Figure 16. The easiest way of locating them is to place your index fingers at the angle of the jaw, just below the ears, and then move them slowly towards the mouth pressing gently against the bone as you do so. At a distance of about one inch from the jaw angle, you should detect identical indentations, on the underside of the bone, the size of a fingertip. Apply pressure to these indentations for two minutes.

If the toothache seems to involve both upper and lower jaws use all three techniques. In addition to pressure point massage, I usually advise my clients to use a traditional folk remedy which nearly always works wonders. Just place a few drops of oil of cloves on the tip of your finger and massage it gently onto the aching tooth and surrounding gum.

But remember that while this treatment eases the discomfort it does nothing to eliminate the underlying cause of the pain which is almost certainly decay and infection. Only your dentist can help you solve the problem once and for all.

Relieving neck pains

Stiffness and discomfort in this area can be caused by a whole host of problems. One of the most common, which results in early morning neck stiffness and general soreness, involves a combination of muscle tension, due to anxiety, and a poor sleeping position which has caused the head to be held awkwardly while you slept. If such stiffness is a recurring problem use the treatment described below together with the stress reduction methods described in Part Four.

The first technique I am going to describe is helpful in relieving almost any sort of neck stiffness, where the symptoms are either difficulty in moving the head from side to side (because the muscles are in spasm) or pain when such a movement is performed.

Sit upright and turn your head as far as is comfortable to the left. Hold your head in your hands, as shown in Figure 17, and attempt to face the front again while resisting the movement with your hands. Keep the pressure steady and move smoothly. Never jerk your neck

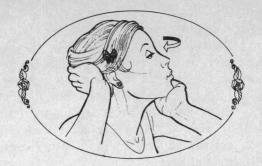

Fig. 17

round. Repeat three times. Next, turn to the right and apply the same sort of resistance while attempting to face the front. Once again do this three times. The effect of the technique is to loosen the muscles and reduce painful tensions. After each resisted head turn you should find that your neck feels less stiff and you are able to move it more easily.

Now I shall describe a squence of techniques which constitute a full treatment for any stiffness in the neck not helped by the method suggested above. People usually find that at the end of these procedures the pain has either gone completely or is far less distressing. You should begin by applying pressure massage.

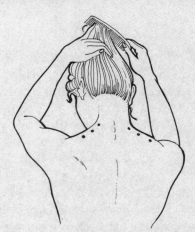

Fig. 18

The points are located at the back of the neck, where it merges with the shoulders. As you explore with your fingertips you should find a number of places especially sensitive to the touch. Apply two minutes firm pressure to each.

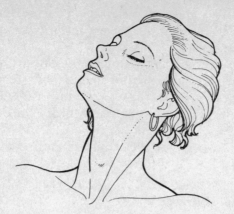

Fig. 19

The next step is to locate the two large muscles either side of the neck. These are the *sternomastoids* as shown in Figure 19 and tension in them can be a source of considerable discomfort. Grasp them using the fingers of both hands. Your fingers should be level with the ear lobes and about three-quarters of an inch behind them. As you turn your head from side to side you will feel the sternomastoids rising up beneath the skin. Give a deep friction massage down the length of these muscles.

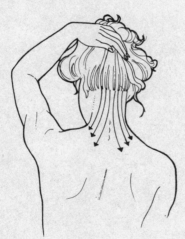

Fig. 20

The final technique in this three-part treatment involves a deep stroking movement using the first two fingers of each hand. Press them firmly against the skin, starting at the base of the skull, and stroke down the neck muscles, maintaining the pressure as shown in Figure 20. Repeat, moving the fingers inwards towards the spine each time you stroke.

Because there are so many underlying causes to this type of difficulty, you will have to experiment with these techniques to find which combinations produce the fastest and most lasting relief. You should also use the prevention exercises which I will describe in Part Three.

From the neck we move to the shoulder, another common area of pain and stiffness.

Relieving shoulder pains

This sequence of massages and movements is especially good for treating a painful condition called 'frozen shoulder', which is caused by an inflammation of the soft tissue around the joint. But it should prove equally effective in easing the discomfort brought about by any kind of shoulder muscle strain.

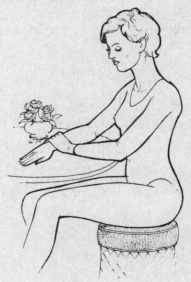

Fig. 21

One:
   Start with a simple isometric exercise. Sitting at a table stretch out the affected arm, and grasp it as shown. Attempt to raise the painful arm while firmly pressing down on it with the other arm for a slow

count of seven. Relax and repeat several times. After each repetition try to raise the arm higher for the next one.

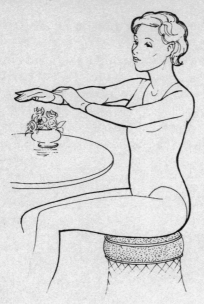

Fig. 22

Two:

Stand up and lean forward from the waist. Let the affected arm hang down, keeping it as limp as you can manage, and begin to make small, circular movements with it. If the arm is really relaxed it should be easy to make it gyrate. Continue to let it swing limply for

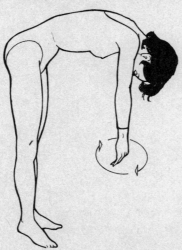

Fig. 23

about 20 seconds. When you feel comfortable in this movement the addition of a small weight (such as an iron) in the hand will make the exercise even more effective.

The final set of treatments consist of deep friction massage applied as follows:

First, massage down the base of the skull and along the shoulder blade following the line in Figure 24a. Next, move onto the breastbone and work under the clavicle from point 'A' following the arrow in Figure 24b.

Now work from point B, at the base of the ribs, up along the side of the ribs until you reach the hollow in front of the shoulder, C.

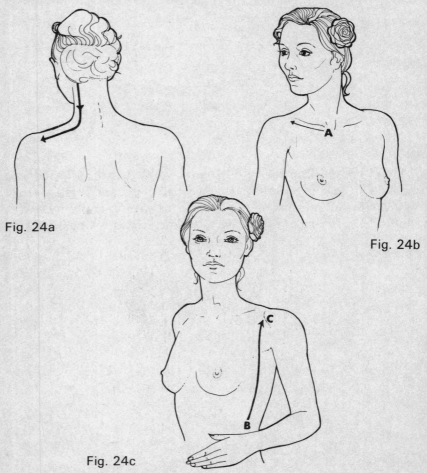

Fig. 24a

Fig. 24b

Fig. 24c

Grasp the muscle on the top of the arm by cupping your hand over it. Lift the muscle, rotate and squeeze it gently several times. Continue this movement halfway down the upper arm. For the last session of deep friction massage you should sit sideways in an upright chair and let your affected arm hang over the back. When you do this you will notice dimples on the shoulder. Apply deep friction massage to these points for twenty seconds each, and finish by massaging along the top and sides of the shoulder for about a minute. Complete the treatment by carrying out one-hand petrissage and effleurage on the sore shoulder. These techniques are described on page 64. You should now find that the pain is greatly eased. In Part Three, I will explain how you can take steps to prevent this type of problem from occurring in the future.

Relieving stomach pains

These can have many causes, some serious, but the majority are no more than a reflection of poor diet or an unwise lifestyle. They may, equally, be the result of psychological difficulties, especially stress, anxiety and emotional upheavals. Check your diet and use the methods I describe in Part Four to reduce everyday tension. If the pains persist consult your doctor.

The treatment here consists of three acupressure techniques which, my experience has shown, can greatly ease the discomfort of an aching stomach. You may be surprised to learn that the first point where pressure must be applied is in the centre of the scalp. This is because acupressure works on energy lines within the body and so has an effect on areas far from the actual point of application. Using Figure 25 you should be able to identify the 'soft spot' shown without much difficulty. Move your fingers forward by about an inch and locate the point of particular tenderness which indicates the correct place to apply firm pressure, with one finger, for two minutes.

You should now locate the following pressure points on the chest and stomach. These are numbered in the drawing as follows:

1: This is located beneath the arm, on the left side of the body, level with the nipple and some two inches away from it.

2: Can be found in the arch of the ribcage just below the breast-bone.

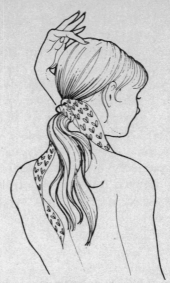

Fig. 25

3: These two points are located each side of the second spot and very close to it.

Apply pressure for two minutes on the first point and one minute on each of the others.

The final pressure point is located beneath the spine a short distance above the crease of the buttocks. Press here for two minutes.

Fig. 26

Relieving travel sickness

There can be few more unpleasant ways to start a holiday or business trip than sickness during your journey. Here is one time when your body certainly makes you take notice of it in a most uncompromising way! Very often my clients ask me if there are some Body Sense techniques which could be used to relieve the misery or better still, prevent the sickness from starting in the first place.

The ancient Chinese took the view that motion illness was mainly a bodily ailment and developed pressure point methods which often prove effective in combating the problem. If you experience even a small amount of discomfort when travelling you should immediately begin to carry out the massage described below. It is much harder to combat the sickness once it has really taken hold, so stay in touch with your body while travelling. Listen to its feelings and be prepared to take prompt action.

Start by locating a point which the Chinese call the 'inside gate'. This point does indeed work as a gate, closing off signals to the 'valve' at the top of the stomach that opens to produce nausea during travel sickness.

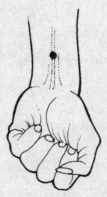

Fig. 27

Make a fist with the left hand. This will cause two tendons, running along the underside of the forearm, to stand out. The point at which you should apply pressure can be found between these tendons some two inches down the wrist fold. Press for ten seconds, release for two seconds, then press again. Repeat half a dozen times then do the same on the right wrist.

Next locate a point on the side of the body just below the ribcage.

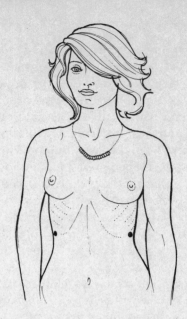

Fig. 28

You can feel this even through clothing. Pressure should be applied firmly and steadily to each side of the body at once. Hold for two *minutes* this time and release.

Finally, press for two minutes on a point located just behind the right knee. It is easier to carry out this massage if you are sitting down.

These techniques will help prevent sickness developing, but you should take sensible precautions as well in order to help your body stay comfortable. Here are six tips which will add to the effectiveness of massage.

* Avoid drinking too much alcohol, especially when flying. Pressurisation in aircraft cabins causes bodily dehydration which alcohol only makes worse. Give yourself plenty of non-alcoholic refreshment, water or still (not fizzy) fruit juices, especially on a long flight.
* Try not to become anxious about the journey. Use the stress control methods I describe in Part Four to help you here.
* Ensure that you get a sufficient rest before a long trip. Do not start out exhausted or your body will be more vulnerable. In Part

Four I will be explaining how you can use Body Sense methods to beat sleepless nights.

* Do not eat rich foods before or during the trip.

* When flying, take off your shoes and loosen any tight clothing. Another effect of the pressurised cabin is to cause certain blood vessels and internal organs to expand. This can produce considerable discomfort if they are restricted by tight garments.

* Choose a sensible place to sit if you are especially susceptible to motion sickness. The centre sections of an aircraft or ship are usually the most stable places. On a boat, stay in the open air as much as possible and avoid areas where the fumes, from engines or galley, are especially strong.

Relieving constipation

An all-too-common complaint, especially in the affluent Western world, constipation produces poisons in the bloodstream which create such problems as headaches, dizziness, shoulder and back pains, insomnia, poor complexion and a loss of energy. The blockage can be brought on by emotional difficulties, excessive stress, lack of exercise and an unsatisfactory diet. If constipation is a recurring health problem then you should start by looking at what you eat. Make certain your diet includes enough raw vegetable and fruit, especially foodstuffs like cabbage, apples, brown rice and bran, which contain fibrous material. Drink plenty of liquids particularly on rising. Then ask yourself whether you take sufficient exercise. An occasional stroll is insufficient to keep a body in good condition, especially when the rest of the day is spent in sedentary activities such as sitting behind a desk. Look at the amount of stress you are being subjected to. Is there too much tension in your everyday life? Take immediate steps to improve any of these situations when they appear to merit attention. Listen to your body. Do not simply try to blast the problem away using increasingly powerful laxatives. Like pain, digestive upsets are often a warning. Your system is sending up a distress signal and you would be foolish to disregard its cry for help.

For relief of constipation, without resort to patent medicines, you should carry out the following Body Sense techniques, but not if you are pregnant or have recently undergone abdominal surgery.

Remember this treatment is only a form of first aid, it will relieve your discomfort but it cannot prevent the problem from recurring. Only you can do that.

Begin by lying on your back, knees bent, and applying gentle pressure to the areas shown in Figure 29.

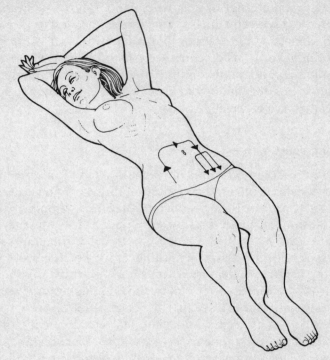

Fig. 29

Use the heel of the hand, or three fingers together in a deep friction movement and move along the body in a clockwise direction. This is actually following the course of a major part of the digestive tract called the colon.

Starting at the lower right hand side of the body move slowly upwards, cross the abdomen just below the navel, and move along the top of the abdomen before descending again on the left side of the body. Pause here and stroke downward for several seconds. Pressure should be steady, but never uncomfortable. If this massage technique causes you any pain you should stop immediately and consult your doctor. Repeat at least six times, more if the discomfort persists.

Stand up for the next exercise, a yoga technique which is especially effective when used together with the massage.

Breathe out as deeply as you are able and bend forward slightly at the waist. Now pull in your stomach as much as possible, without causing yourself any discomfort, and perform a 'pumping' action with the muscles of the abdomen. This is achieved by moving your stomach briskly in and out, making it travel as far as you can in each direction. Hold your breath while doing this and carry on for as long as it is comfortable to do so. When you need to inhale again, stop the pumping, straighten up and breathe in. Take a rest and then repeat the exercise. Do this a total of four times.

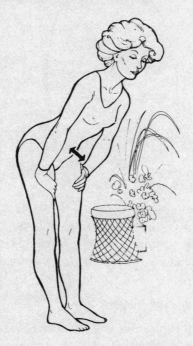

Fig. 30

We now move to acupressure, starting on a point located exactly halfway between the navel and a line marking the join between leg and body – marked (A) in Figure 31. Use one finger to apply a steady pressure to this point for two minutes.

Next find the point marked (B) on the diagram. This lies directly above (A) about halfway between the navel and the right nipple. Once again apply firm, single-finger pressure for two minutes.

These are key releasing points for intestinal blockages and should produce rapid relief from the discomfort.

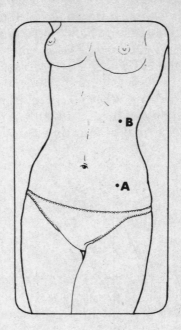

Fig. 31

Following this treatment, constipation will usually clear up quickly. But I do stress, once again, the need to see this condition not as an uncomfortable nuisance, but as a warning from the body that some aspect of your current lifestyle needs changing.

Relieving pain in arms and hands

I have grouped these under one treatment heading, because a single sequence of massages should alleviate pain in any part of the arm. The painful conditions immediately helped by these techniques include tennis and golfer's elbows, familiar problems for many sportsmen and women – and perhaps for you too!

Sit comfortably in front of a table with your aching arm resting on a pillow. Begin with about 20 seconds effleurage on the whole arm. Follow this by petrissage. You can learn about these two basic massage methods by turning to pages 64 and 65.

Now carry out a deep friction massage, circling around the wrist. When you reach the protruding bone on the outside top edge of the wrist, perform deep friction around this too. Then proceed as follows:

One:

Pull the wrist gently outwards and release.

Two:

Carry out deep friction massage in the grooves on the back of the hands, working from web of skin between the fingers towards the wrist.

Three:

Apply deep friction to each finger in turn, working from the tip to the base. As you reach the end of the finger give it a gentle pull.

Four:

Apply a final session of deep friction to the muscular pads at the base of the thumb and little finger.

Continue the treatment by making a fist with the painful hand and bending back the wrist. This should cause several muscles to rise noticeably along the forearm forming grooves. Even if these grooves do not become clearly visible, it will still be possible to locate them by touch.

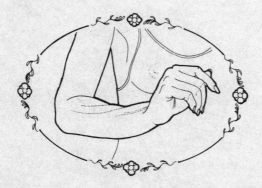

Fig. 32

Place your 1st and 2nd fingers in the groove at the wrist end, apply deep friction concentrating on any painful areas. Move your fingers about a quarter-of-an-inch and repeat. Continue in this way until you arrive at the elbow and work around it searching for painful spots. Now continue up the arm for about 3 inches above the elbow. Go back to the wrist and repeat this procedure along the other grooves between the muscles. Do one handed petrissage along the forearm and upper arm. Complete the massage with effleurage.

Relieving back pains

These are among the most common problems I am asked to treat. Research has shown that in the Western world more than 80% of us will suffer from some sort of back trouble during our lives. One theory is that this is the price we pay for walking on two legs, and this pain has the distinction of being the single greatest cause of lost working days. But it is an area of difficulty where Body Sense Therapy can offer fast relief from discomfort and the hope of permanent prevention. I will deal with ways of avoiding trouble in

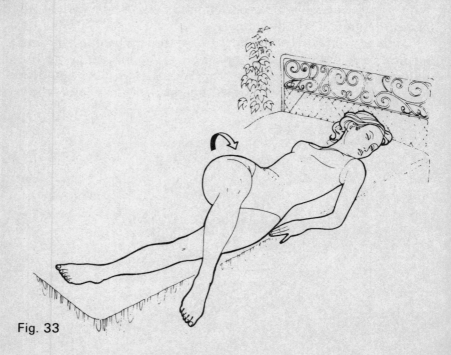

Fig. 33

the next part of the book. Here I want to describe a short, successful form of treatment that you can use any time back pains strike. Since the vast majority of discomfort occurs in the lower back, between the base of the ribs and the tail bone at the bottom of the spine, this is the area I will concentrate on here.

The first movement is derived from a technique used with such success by American chiropractors that it earns them a considerable fortune each year, in fact it is known in the profession as the million dollar roll! Carry out the movements on both sides of the body regardless of the exact location of the lower back pain.

Lie on a bed on your back close to the left side and cross your right leg over the left. The crossover point must be well above the left knee. As you move the right leg it will raise the hip which now points towards the ceiling.

With your upper back and right shoulder held flat against the bed, push your hip forwards half-a-dozen times. Keep the movement smooth and gentle. This hip push should be performed with a rotating action that induces a feeling of stretch across the whole of the back, while bringing the right foot closer to the floor. Unless both movements occur the technique is not being carried out correctly.

Try to remain relaxed throughout the exercise. If you have any difficulty in keeping your right shoulder flat against the bed, or if it has a tendency to rise with the hip, try stretching out your right arm and, if the bed is narrow enough, grasping the other side.

After performing this movement continuously for about 20 seconds, reverse your position so that the left leg now crosses the right in exactly the same way as before, and repeat.

Now bend the knee on the most painful side and clasp it as close to the same shoulder as possible. Your heel should be close to the buttock. Hold this for at least 30 seconds and slowly straighten the leg, bringing it back to the bed. Finally, lie on your back and try to lengthen each leg in turn as much as possible.

Relieving upper leg pains

These are due to pain signals travelling along the sciatic nerve which runs closest to the surface at the highest point of the buttocks. From there it passes into the back of the thigh where it supplies the hamstring muscles. Pain along this pathway may be more acute when you are especially fatigued or during damp weather.

A good starting point for tackling discomfort in the legs is to perform deep friction massage in the naturally occurring dimples at the base of the spine. To locate them, push the buttocks together. The dimples can then be seen, using a mirror, or identified by touch. After massaging this area, move your fingers gradually downwards searching out any other small indentations which feel painful to the touch. Apply deep friction to each.

You should also check the crease under the fold of the buttocks because, if the ligaments are strained, there will be painful spots here as well. Now carry out deep friction massage with the heel of the hand working diagonally across the buttocks from the lowest central point outwards to the hips.

Further relief can be achieved through stretching the sciatic nerve. Start by sitting upright on the floor. Then pull up from the base of the spine to make sure your back is straight with your legs stretched out in front, feet turned slightly outwards. Sit tall with your spine *straight* and the leg muscles as relaxed as possible. Do a series of gentle forward pushes from the base of the spine.

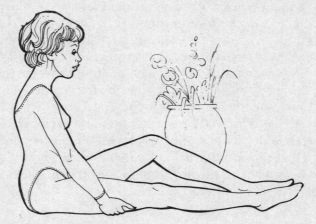

Fig. 34

This movement stretches the nerves and muscles at the back of the legs together. Now bend the knee a little on the side which is not painful in order to increase the stretch on the afflicted leg.

Continue with effleurage to the backs of the thighs and buttocks until such time as the whole area feels warmer. Lift and knead the muscles with a petrissage movement. Finish off by rolling the thigh muscles vigorously between the hands.

Relieving knee pain

This can be due to a number of causes, some relatively trivial others important enough to deserve professional treatment. If you suffer from chronic knee pain seek advice from your doctor. The techniques described for this treatment do not provide any kind of a cure for the underlying conditions, but they are often effective in relieving the pain.

In most cases the large muscles on the top and inside of the thigh are involved in this condition and must be included in the massage. Begin by working on these important muscles with effleurage, one hand after the other along the top of the thigh, starting at the knee and working towards the groin. Repeat on the inside and outside of the thigh.

Now, starting at the knee, do petrissage along the top and inner side of the thigh, working as before from the knee to the groin. Details of this massage technique will be found on page 65.

Stroke the area around the knee, using both hands, one following the other in a circular motion. Continue for 30 seconds.

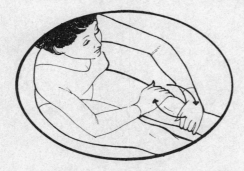

Fig. 35

Follow this with a deep friction massage, circling around the knee and using the tips of the middle fingers. Start at the outside, as shown in Figure 36 and, when you reach the inside of the knee, continue doing deep friction down the inside of the lower leg for a distance of about one inch.

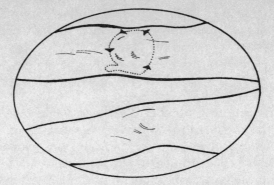

Fig. 36

Massage back up to the knee and continue with deep friction until you complete the circle. Carry on in the same way down the outside of the knee and into the space behind the knee. Pause there to carry out 15 seconds deep friction in the one spot.

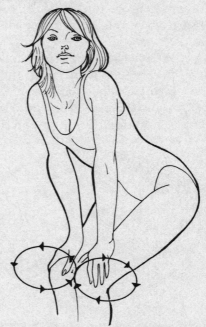

Fig. 37

Loosen the muscles by standing up and placing your hands just above the knees, feet together. Perform a sideways figure of eight.

By following this simple course of treatment you should be able to ease knee pains considerably after only a few minutes' work.

Relieving lower leg pains

An important cause of pain in the lower legs is a condition known as *shin splints* which is brought about through excessive flexing of the foot. It is likely to occur whenever a person who is out of condition engages in vigorous activity and works the feet harder than untrained muscles can tolerate. Shin splints are also frequently found among women who wear high heels. In this case the only sensible course of action is to switch to flat shoes for a few weeks while easing the discomfort using the techniques I shall describe.

Start with deep friction massage along a groove in the leg which follows the line of the shinbone down the outside of the leg.

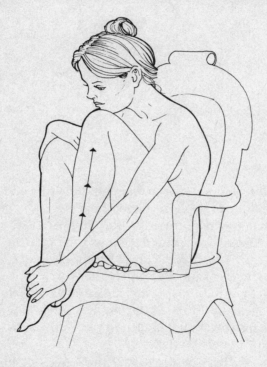

Fig. 38

Work upwards from ankle to knee massaging with the first and second fingers. Repeat five times.

Now, using the heel of the hand, apply firm pressure with deep friction to the large muscle that lies beside the shinbone. Start at the ankle, as before, press steadily, move your hand a short distance further up the muscle and repeat. Stop when you reach the knee and repeat the whole massage five times.

If your calf muscles are painful apply effleurage on the area from ankle to knee, stroking with one hand after the other. Follow with two-handed petrissage starting behind the ankle, moving up the achilles tendon, and working upwards to the knee. For details of these techniques turn to page 64 and 65. Now place the heels of the hands on each side of the calf muscle and shake it vigorously rolling the muscle between your hands. Finish as always with effleurage.

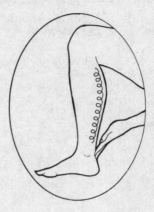

Fig. 39

The final technique eases pain in both the shin and calf. Get hold of a large book, a telephone directory is ideal, and stand on it with your feet hanging over the edge. Keeping the knees straight, lower your heels towards the ground as far as you can without overbalancing. This gently stretches the lower leg muscles and soothes away the pain-producing tension. Repeat six times.

This treatment should bring about rapid relief from the discomfort caused by lower leg pains. But for lasting freedom from such problems you should take the preventative actions described in the next part of this book.

As with all the conditions and methods of pain relief I have described here, it is never enough just to treat the symptoms. One must always seek out the cause of the discomfort and work to eliminate this as well.

Cold hands and feet

If you suffer from cold hands and feet try this technique to improve your circulation.

Lie down on your back and lift your arms and legs straight up in the air in front of you. Shake and vibrate them as rapidly as possible, continuing until you feel warmth in your extremities.

I must end this part with the warning given at the start. Do not disregard pain or merely try to get rid of symptoms. Pain is a signal from your body that something has gone wrong, take notice of that message and seek professional advice if it persists.

PART TWO

Your health-giving hands

In creating the Body Sense way to health I have brought together methods of massage and movement from all parts of the world and many different periods of history. Some originated in ancient Chinese and Indian therapies and have proved their health enhancing powers down the centuries. Others I have developed from the discoveries of modern researchers in the clinics and universities of Europe and America. Many have evolved from my practical experiences in helping my clients to enjoy full and lasting fitness and from that deep, almost instinctive knowledge of the human body which professional dancers come to possess. Although very different in their origins, each of these techniques shares one essential feature. They draw their potency and exert their effect not from any external agency but by harnessing directly the natural health giving forces within the human body. They gently help you to peak mental and physical condition by taking advantage of the regenerative powers of muscle and nerve that have gradually evolved down the long history of mankind's development.

The value of different forms of massage has been recognised for thousands of years. Although often neglected by Western physicians, its powerful physical and psychological benefits are now, slowly, being recognised by orthodox medicine. Massage is one of the most basic forms of self-treatment we possess and an instant response to pain which comes naturally to even the smallest child. What does a toddler do after taking a tumble or a knock, apart from bawling the house down? Almost always he tries to soothe away the discomfort by rubbing the afflicted body area.

In essence that is all there is to massage. A return to the childhood reaction to rub something better. But your health-giving hands are capable of more than simply easing a physical pain. They can actually promote permanent well-being by enabling the body to work more efficiently. The secret lies in knowing exactly where and how to use the healing touch. There is nothing mystical or mysterious about any of this knowledge, nor do you need to be a specially gifted person to make use of it. Each one of us possess these powers and can learn how to perfect them quickly and easily.

I have stressed the fact that Body Sense Therapy allows you to keep *yourself* in peak condition without the need for any help. This may strike you as rather strange because massage is normally thought of as something which has to be done *for you* by another person. In the past this has certainly been true and, to my mind, was always the main difficulty about using the technique successfully. I remember, several years ago, one of my film actress clients raising that very point when she told me: 'I feel marvellous after a massage, but you are never around to give me one when I most need it!' Her view was echoed by others and led me to create a system of massage which people might alleviate pain, eliminate tensions and restore their bodies to health. I will tell you how to use these self-massage methods on yourself at any time you feel the need for a mental or physical boost; before starting for home after a hard day in the office, for example, after driving through heavy traffic, when too tired to sleep properly, or in order to ease away an unexpected ache or niggling pain. The only body present need be your own and the restorative powers of this health giving procedure are never any further away than your fingertips. I want to tell you how to set about performing a massage, first by offering some general advice and then by describing in detail the techniques for carrying out a number of basic massage movements.

How to start

The massage sessions will be easier and more pleasant if you use a lubricant to help your hands slide smoothly and silkily across the skin. Although some people use powder, I favour a vegetable oil: coconut has the advantage of being light and easy to remove afterwards, but soya, sunflower and almond oils are equally good.

My personal preference is to perfume the chosen lubricant by the addition of a few drops of what are called *essential oils*. These are the concentrated nectars of flowers or plants and not only give the preparation an attractive scent but, because they are one of the few substances which can be completely absorbed through the skin, are directly beneficial to the body. Where a client is suffering from muscle tenderness due to overexertion, from playing a sport or digging the garden for example, I would advise the addition of sage oil. This is also beneficial for alleviating rheumatic pains or inflammation. Two favourites of mine, camomile and lavender, are especially good when massaging to relieve a headache, while lemon grass is excellent for toning and stimulating the muscles.

Vegetable oils can be purchased in any supermarket or health food store, while essential oils may be obtained from herb suppliers or most large pharmacies. Mix them by stirring in approximately eight drops of essential oil to each cupful of vegetable oil. The exact proportions are a matter of personal taste. Experiment when you first start, keeping a note of the different mixes used, until you find one that best suits your needs.

Making an aromatic soother

On the subject of essential oils, the following aromatic soother is one of the most pleasant and effective means I know for dealing with sore muscles. It consists of a ball of paraffin wax, scented with oils, which can be rubbed over the aching area. The result is a pleasant, comforting sensation of warmth which quickly eases away the hurt. But use an aromatic soother only when relieving soreness in the muscles. It should not be rubbed over inflamed spots or places where the skin is broken. You create the soother like this:

Ingredients: 1 cake of paraffin wax; 15 drops oil of camphor; 15 drops wintergreen oil; 5 drops oil of rosemary.

Mixing method; Melt the wax in a small metal container standing in a large pot of boiling water. When melted, gradually mix in the three essential oils, stirring with a wooden spoon. Now allow it to cool. When the wax has reached the stage of being almost solid, remove it from the pot and mould it into balls each one about the size of your palm. Wrap in waxed paper or tin foil and store in a suitable container. Aromatic soothers are especially helpful in the treatment of aches due to sporting activity, gardening, or any unusually demanding muscle work. Their effect is somewhat like that of a liniment but they are far more relaxing.

Though helpful and pleasant to use, oils are certainly not essential in order to use self-massage techniques to relieve stress, ease tensions or eliminate a sudden pain. But if you are settling down to a more prolonged massage session, where there is the time and privacy to carry out a complete course of Body Sense Therapy, then I strongly advise the use of oils as part of your regular massage procedure.

Positions for self-massage

One:

For neck and upper back sit at a table, bend your head toward and support it on a small cushion.

Two:

For the lower back lie on the floor and place a cushion under your head and shoulders. If you now bend your knees you should be able to reach the lower back easily by sliding your hands under your waist.

Three:

For stomach massage remain on the floor, in the position described in *Two*.

Four:

For the sides of the lower back remain on the floor and turn on one side. Massage can be performed on other areas of the body without difficulty when sitting, standing or lying.

Before you start, warm your hands by rubbing them together for a few seconds and then shaking them, as if getting rid of water. This brings the blood to fingers and palms. It also 'charges' the hands since the orientals tell us that the right hand (yang) is positive and the left hand (yin) is negative. When applying massage try to mould your hands to the shape of the body beneath them. Keep the speed and rhythm consistent throughout and start and finish each treatment using the smooth, stroking movement called *effleurage* which I shall describe in a moment.

The ancient Chinese regarded the stomach as the seat of bodily power and recommended that massage should be from this area. They performed many activities designed to take advantage of the power of the stomach and transmit it to the furthest reaches of the body. In massage all you have to do to achieve this goal is to tense the stomach muscles slightly when carrying out the movements. At the same time relax your hands so that power radiates from the stomach. This combination of relaxed hands and tense stomach ensures that you do not pinch or grip yourself too hard.

If you have a painful joint or a muscle which is too sore to massage, work above and below the area to start with, gradually moving closer and closer to the painful spot as the tenderness decreases.

How to massage

The techniques I am about to describe will be used over and over again throughout the book, to enhance health, alleviate problems caused by stress and tension, improve your appearance and relieve a wide range of pains. There is no need to try and learn them all at once – they will come quite easily with practice. But I do suggest that you read quickly through each one so as to grasp the general idea behind them. They are all straightforward and you will soon become an expert in their use.

Effleurage

The name comes from the French *effleurer* meaning to 'skim over' and it is a very apt description of the technique, involving as it does a stroking movement in which pressure is firm on the *upward* strokes and light on the return strokes. By upwards I mean in *the direction of the heart*, no matter on which part of the body it is being performed.

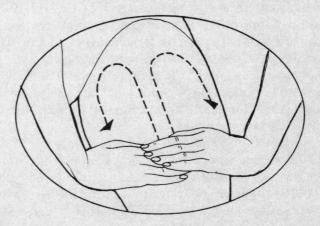

Fig. 40

Effleurage can be carried out using both hands together, or one hand after the other. When massaging smaller areas it may be performed with the finger-tips. At all times the movements must be smooth and regular. Figure 40 shows the way two handed effleurage is performed.

Petrissage

This is another word taken from the French, and means 'to knead'. It refers to a movement carried out by pressing muscles firmly against their underlying bones, with the palm of the hand, sliding the hand forward a couple of inches and then picking up the muscle with the fingers and thumb, giving a gentle squeeze as you do so. This can be done by one hand in a continuous movement or with each hand in turn. Keep your fingers relaxed throughout so as to prevent pinching the skin.

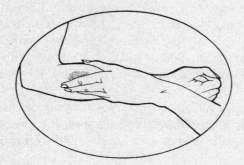

Fig. 41

Deep friction massage

This is carried out by making small, circular movements with one or more fingers pressed firmly against the muscle. As the fingers are rotated it is important not to let them slide across the skin which

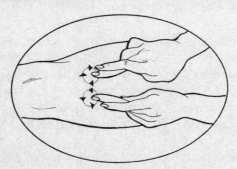

Fig. 42

should move with the fingers. After making a few circles in one spot, shift to another location about a quarter inch away and repeat the movements. You should continue to use deep friction massage down the length of the sore muscle.

Vibrating

Press one or more fingers firmly against the skin and vibrate the hand as rapidly as possible. When doing this it helps to tense your forearm muscles as though lifting a heavy load.

Acupressure

More than 4000 years ago Chinese physicians observed that, when people were sick, it was quite common to find points of special soreness on different parts of the body, often in areas a long way away from the apparent cause of the illness. They also found that pressure on these points relieved pain and helped to cure the complaint. Over a period of many years, they mapped the precise location of more than 1000 of these acupressure points, developing their observations into a systematic and extremely effective form of treatment.

Acupressure specialists say that, when we are diseased, the flow of vital energy through the body is disrupted. Pressure on the correct points starts this flowing smoothly again and so restores the patient to health.

One of the main difficulties confronting non-specialists when they try to make use of the same technique is locating the exact pressure points. Few books on the subject do more than provide illustrations showing their general position and, since the precise location of each varies between one individual and another, such drawings are of little practical help.

I have found two infallible methods for putting your finger, literally, on the correct spot. The first is by the look or feel of the skin. Almost all the points are located in a small depression which is easy to detect. The second is determined by the body's response to touch. These points are always *more tender* than the surrounding area of skin, something which becomes immediately obvious when you apply a little pressure.

When acupressure is the right technique to use, I will show you the general location of the pressure points and you can then find the exact spots using the two clues of appearance and tenderness.

In acupressure massage you apply a fixed amount of pressure to the skin for periods of time ranging from a few seconds up to two minutes. I will tell you how long to maintain the pressure when describing a particular technique, but the force should remain constant at 10 lbs. The best way to teach yourself how to apply this amount of pressure is to practise with bathroom scales. Using one finger, depress the platform until the pointer moves to the 10 lb mark. Feel the amount of force necessary to achieve this deflection. Repeat the same exercise a number of times until you are able to move the pointer to 10 lbs with your eyes closed.

Here, then, are the basic massage techniques you will be using. They are perfectly safe provided you carry them out as I describe. Do not attempt any form of massage, however, if you are recovering from a serious illness or operation, or are running a temperature. Do not massage any part of your body where varicose veins or skin irritations are present. If you are pregnant, avoid using any stomach massage, and the same applies if you have just had abdominal surgery. Other types of surgery may make it unwise to massage certain parts of the body and you should take medical advice before doing so. Indeed the most sensible course of action before embarking on any self-help health programme, is to seek medical advice should you have the slightest doubt about the wisdom of what you are doing.

Because it is impossible to achieve good health while suffering from any aches or pains, especially when these are persistent, the first step may be to alleviate the discomfort they cause. This can usually be done by making use of the wide range of techniques already described and which can be applied whenever life is being made miserable because of headache, muscle stiffness, poor digestion or some other similar ailments.

PART THREE

The Body Sense way to pain-free living

I am sure you are familiar with the old saying about prevention being better than cure. If only more people would turn those wise words into everyday deeds where their health is concerned, there would be a transformation in the nation's mental and physical fitness. While many of the essentials of a healthy life are well known they are seldom widely adopted. We tend to spend more time talking about the value of a sensible diet, regular exercise, clean air and proper sleep than doing anything about it!

But there is another equally valuable, though seldom appreciated, means by which you can help yourself to health. In Part One I described ways in which common discomforts such as headaches, muscle stiffness and digestion problems could be relieved *after* they had arisen. It is, of course, far better for one's health to prevent these debilitating aches and pains from occurring in the first place. In this part of the book I will tell you how to do just that.

Even if you feel well and fit at the moment, it may still be harder than it once was to carry out certain actions or perform particular movements. I do not mean strenuous activities such as jogging or lifting heavy weights, but rather the kind of everyday tasks which can normally be accomplished without difficulty: reaching for a high shelf, for example, lifting something without back strain, turning to look over your shoulder or walking some distance without effort. If movements as commonplace as these produce a sensation of stiffness, a feeling of mild discomfort or a twinge of real pain, then your body is protesting. The system is not working as well as it should and you must take prompt action to put things right.

The trouble is that, especially when you are busy, such minor messages tend to get overlooked or dismissed as part of the penalty of 'growing old'. What is more, because your body is very clever at discovering new ways of doing things that avoid the discomforting movements, you may not even be aware any difficulties exist. Even after Body Sense training it is still possible to miss these early warning messages. To help overcome the problem I have devised a series of ten simple exercises which allow you to become immediately aware of potential danger spots around the body. I call this my Awareness Analysis, and it consists of the kind of movements I would ask a client to carry out during my initial examination, while I am planning the best programme to help them back to peak condition. By performing the Analysis for yourself you will be able to assess the efficiency with which all the major muscle groups are functioning. Analysis will also direct you to the most appropriate Body Sense Therapy methods for combating any problems which do come to light and show you how to use these in the most effective order by assigning a priority to each trouble spot.

If you are able to carry out all the exercises without effort, it indicates that your body is working well. But you must not become too complacent. Good health cannot be stored up like power in a battery. The price of fitness is constant vigilance and sensible exercise. To remain healthy it is essential to stay in touch with your body using sixth sense training and by carrying out this Analysis at least once a month – it only takes five minutes – so as to monitor the efficiency with which your muscles are working.

Awareness Analysis

I am going to ask you to do ten non-stressful exercises and then score the results. In one or two cases I will tell you exactly what score to award. In most instances, however, you will have to give yourself marks on your subjective assessment of how easy it was to carry out the required movements.

For any that are performed without any stiffness, discomfort or undue effort, the score is always zero. If they could not be performed at all because the muscles were too stiff or it was too painful to proceed then score 10 points.

Between these extremes give yourself points according to any problems experienced. The harder it was the higher the score. By using this simple system of marking it becomes possible for you to rank each of the exercises in order of difficulty and so discover which parts of the body are in most urgent need to help. Choose a time of day when you can be alone for at least five minutes. Loosen any tight clothing and take off your shoes. Now proceed as follows:

Exercise One: NECK. Look first to the left and then to the right. Turn your head as far as you can without serious discomfort. An effortless 90° turn in each direction produces a zero score. If you were unable to look in either direction without stiffness or pain award 10 points. Give a score between these two depending on the amount of head turn possible and the degree of discomfort experienced. Note whether it was more difficult to turn your head in one direction than the other.

Exercise Two: NECK. Tilt your head forward and rotate it in a circle, first in a clockwise then an anticlockwise direction. Try to complete a full turn in each direction, stretching your neck muscles enough to bring the side of the head as close to the shoulders as you can. When this is done there may be, in addition to some stiffness or pain, a noticeable clicking sound. As for the head turning exercise, score zero for an effortless rotation; the inability to turn your head as described would be worth 10 points.

Exercise Three: SHOULDER. Stand upright and attempt to touch the tips of your fingers behind your back, as shown in Figure 43.

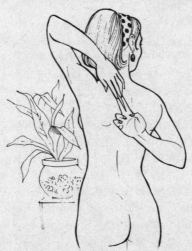

Fig. 43

There is no score if this can be done easily. If the fingers are almost touching (look in a mirror when in doubt) then give yourself 5 points. If the hands are widely separated this scores 10 points.

Exercise Four: UPPER BACK. Lie face down on the floor with a pillow under your stomach, hands at your sides. Keeping the lower part of your body flat on the ground, try to lift your upper back and shoulders without any help with your arms. If you can keep your body raised for ten seconds there is no score. Five seconds gives a score of 5 points, while there is a 10 point score for anything less than five seconds.

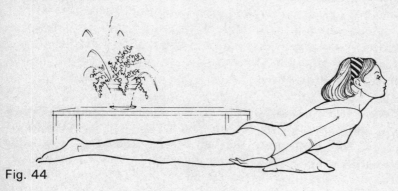

Fig. 44

Exercise Five: LOWER BACK. Lie face down again, but this time without the pillow. Place your hands, palm upwards, under your thighs. Keeping your legs straight, raise them as high as you can and count how long they remain raised, stopping at 10 seconds. If you managed the full time without effort or pain there is no score. As above, award 5 points for a five second raise and 10 for anything less.

Exercise Six: STOMACH. Lie on your back, hands behind your head, knees bent up as far as possible and feet flat on the ground. Without moving or lifting your legs, attempt to touch your elbows to your knees. You only need to do this movement once. If you found no difficulty, there is no score. If you were unable to do it at all, award 10 points. Score between these in the usual way.

Exercise Seven: WRISTS. All I want you to do here is stretch out your arm and rotate the wrists, one after the other, first in a clockwise then an anticlockwise direction. Notice any stiffness or discomfort and score as before according to difficulty.

Exercise Eight: UPPER LEGS AND KNEES. Stand with your feet about twelve inches apart and try to place your palms flat on the floor between them, *without* bending at the knee. Score according to the ease or difficulty with which this can be done.

Exercise Nine: LOWER LEGS. Rise onto the balls of your feet (not halfway) and, keeping your legs straight, walk around the room. Try to do this for 30 seconds, but make a mental note of how long it is before your muscles seem tired or become stiff. There is no score if you manage the full half minute without difficulty. If you experienced the first twinge of discomfort at about 15 seconds then score 5 points. If you were unable to remain on your toes for the full 30 seconds score 10 points.

Exercise Ten: ANKLES. Stand straight and rest your right hand on a chair or table for balance. Now lift your left leg as high as possible, at the same time rising onto the ball of your right foot. Hold this position for a slow count to three and then bring your heel slowly back to the floor, lowering the left leg as you do so. Next extend the left leg out to the side, once again raising yourself up onto the ball of the foot. Count to three and lower yourself as before. Finally extend the leg as far as possible behind your body. Repeat all three movements using the right leg. If you can do all these without discomfort or stiffness there is no score. Otherwise award points, as in each of the other exercises, on the basis of difficulty.

How the Analysis helps

In just about five minutes you have analysed the functioning of most of the body's major muscle groups. For peak health they should all be in a good enough condition to allow the exercises to be completed easily and effortlessly. The chart below enables you to record your score for each and find out which of the Body Sense techniques is best suited to your particular needs. You will probably find it helpful to use this chart on a number of occasions, as you make the Analysis a part of your regular health check programme, so I advise you to copy it out onto a sheet of paper.

In the fourth column, headed 'Priority' you should rank each of the scores, from highest to lowest. Identical scores are given an equal ranking. This tells you the *order* in which to carry out the appropriate techniques listed in the column headed 'What I Can Do To Help Myself'. Start with those exercises that received the highest score and work your way down the list. Zero score items can be ignored. Each of the techniques I describe has a *time required* for completion noted against it. This is the *average* needed to carry out a particular pain prevention method, based on my experience with many clients. You should not worry, however, if it takes you a little longer than I suggest to complete the procedure, especially when you

Awareness Analysis Chart

Exercise	Part of Body Involved	Score	Priority	What I Can Do To Help Myself?
One Two	Neck			Indian dancer's head movements
Three	Shoulder			The Circle The Shrug The Shimmy
Four Five	Upper & Lower Back			The Pelvic Tilt & Lift The Lower Back Limber The Spine Stretch and Relax The Hip Limber The Cobra
Six	Stomach			The Knees-up/Sit-Up The Double Leg Lift
Seven	Wrists			Heun-Sau
Eight	Upper legs and knee			The Ballet Bend & Reach Jazz Dancers Leg Swing Full Plié
Nine	Lower Legs			The Toe Point
Ten	Ankles			The Demiplié Zenutsu Dachi

first start. The times should also be considered a minimum. You may find it beneficial to carry out a particular technique several times each day, and one can do so perfectly safely.

I have included the times because most people prefer to create their own individual health care programmes which have to be slotted into whatever free moments they have available.

After ranking your score you should turn to the first technique indicated and start working to restore muscle efficiency and prevent pain.

Indian dancer's head movements: TIME REQUIRED: 30 SECONDS. This is a technique to improve the suppleness and strength of neck muscles which has been taught for many thousands of years to Hindu temple dancers. If you have ever had the pleasure of watching these slender, graceful girls perform you will be well aware how effortless their head movements are. With only a little practice the same degree of suppleness can be yours. This will not only ensure you are able to move your head freely, without the slightest trace of stiffness or twinges of pain, but help to create and preserve a youthful appearance, by enhancing the muscle tone of the neck and chin.

Stand upright and move your head forward, and backwards, keeping your chin parallel to the ground. Another way of making sure your head position is right is to imagine that the line in Figure 45 is a rod which passes through your skull. As you perform the movements keep the rod exactly at right angles to the ground.

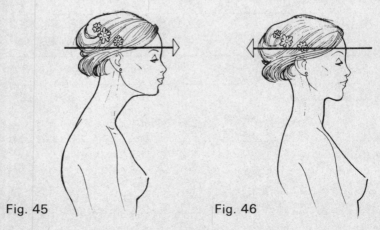

Fig. 45   Fig. 46

This completes the first sequence of movements. The head goes forward, returns to the normal position and is then drawn back. The next step is to move it from side to side. As before, imagine the vertical rod at right angles to the ground, and your chin parallel to the ground. At first it will probably help to practise before a mirror. As you will now be aware, the full sequence involves moving your head forward, returning to the starting position and bringing the head back. Return to the starting position and move the head to the left, return and move to the right. I suggest you start with three repetitions of the complete sequence building up, over a period of time, to ten repetitions.

While carrying out these movements keep your body as relaxed as possible and avoid jerking the neck. Complete each sequence by tilting your head first to the left, then to the right before finally performing a gentle circling movement in both a clockwise and anticlockwise direction. Allow the neck to relax while circling so that it almost feels as if your head is about to drop off. After only a short amount of time you will start to enjoy the benefits of this exercise. Stiffness during movement will disappear, muscles will regain lost tone and aging flabbiness will be reduced. You will support your head without needless tension, so reducing the likelihood of headaches, You are also likely to feel brighter and more alert as your brain responds to the enhanced circulation. Use these exercises to safeguard your health at times when it is more than usually probable that you will place unnatural strain on the neck muscles, for instance following a long drive or air journey.

Shoulders: The Circle – TIME REQUIRED: 1 MINUTE. While sitting or standing I want you to slowly circle your shoulders. Bring them up as far as you can towards your ears. Now move them forward, then down and finally back to the starting position so they have travelled in a complete circle. Repeat in the opposite direction. Spend 30 seconds circling your shoulders in a clockwise direction and another 30 seconds moving them anticlockwise. When you become used to this exercise try rotating the shoulders alternately so that the movement is fluid and rythmical.

The Shrug: TIME REQUIRED: 30 SECONDS. All I want you to do here is shrug your shoulders. It sounds too simple to be of much help, but experience has shown that this movement works wonders for stiffness. Lift them as high as you can before allowing them to drop back again.

The Shimmy: TIME REQUIRED: 30 SECONDS. This is a movement I have adapted from the Belly Dancer's famous routine, but it is equally helpful to non-dancers. It is a particularly good movement for loosening the shoulders and toning up the muscles.

Stand or sit comfortably, with your hands hanging relaxed at your side. Start by swinging each shoulder backwards and forwards as shown in Figure 47.

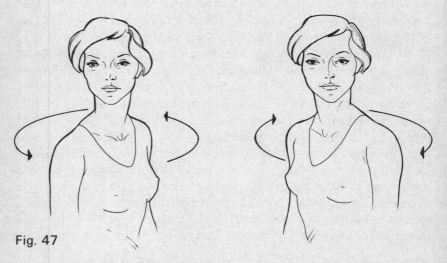

Fig. 47

Your neck should be thought of as a pivot around which the shoulders swing too and fro.

Swing your shoulders slowly at first and increase speed gradually. Keep the movements smooth and try to relax the rest of your body, especially your arms and hands which should not be allowed to swing freely. As you speed up, your shoulders should start to 'shimmy'.

Picture a dog which has just finished a swim and is busily shaking the water off his coat. Hold this image in mind and try to imitate it. You may find this a bit tricky at first, but it will come with a little practice. Mastering the 'shimmy' technique is well worth the time involved because it works wonders for stiff shoulders and greatly enhances suppleness in all the muscle groups. This movement should be done for 30 seconds.

Finish the sequence by standing with your feet apart and hands clasped behind your back. Now bend forward at the waist raising your arms as high as possible behind you.

For maximum suppleness and freedom from shoulder discomfort you should carry out all these movements at least once a day, they only take a total of three minutes to complete. Perform them slowly at first, increasing speed as your muscles become freer and start working more efficiently.

Tennis Elbow: TIME REQUIRED: 3 MINUTES. You don't have to play tennis to develop tennis elbow. It can affect golfers, fishermen, violinists, even housewives. This is a good preventive exercise. Rest your forearm on a table, palm facing upwards. Hold in your hand a 3–5 lbs weight, such as a small book. Bend and lower your forearm several times until it feels tired. Repeat with the weight facing away from you. Try also gently squeezing a small object such as a ball of putty or plasticine in your hand to tone the muscles.

Upper Back/Lower Back: TOTAL TIME REQUIRED: 3 MINUTES. The few minutes spent carrying out the Body Sense exercises for back pains could not be used more wisely. As I mentioned earlier, back problems are among the most widespread ailments which afflict mankind and you should take early warnings of trouble very seriously indeed.

My clients often ask why they should start to suffer from this kind of problem after a lifetime of freedom from discomfort. Back pains, like neck stiffness and 'frozen shoulder' are difficulties associated with middle age that cannot normally be traced to any particular event or accident. Rather they have to be considered as the inevitable consequence of decades of poor posture, inadequate muscle tone, incorrect movements and lack of proper exercise. With age, the once supple ligaments joining muscles to bones begin to harden or ossify. The deterioration starts around the age of thirty, but may not become noticeable for up to twenty years. From the age of twenty, however, there has usually been a decrease in the efficiency of blood circulation through the muscles. Denied the levels of oxygen and nutrition needed for healthy growth and function, they become weaker and less able to withstand life's stresses. Those whose task it is to support the spine gradually decline in effectiveness, the bones move out of alignment and press on the nerves which pass through them on their way to the brain, thus causing pain. Therefore, by strengthening the *muscles* and paying attention to posture, you can achieve perfect skeletal support.

Whatever your age, it will help you to perform these two exercises regularly and monitor your back muscles, using the Assessment Analysis, at frequent intervals. Even if you have been free from trouble up to now, take notice of any twinges felt when you carried out the Analysis as it is extremely foolish to ignore such messages. Some kinds of back problems, when fully developed, are difficult to treat successfully.

Incidentally, back problems do not suddenly arise from a single movement. You often hear people say they were just bending down to tie their shoe lace (or some other innocuous movement) when their back went out. You can be sure, however, that their problem developed over years of accumulated abuse. That sudden movement was simply the last straw!

As posture is so important in the prevention of all types of back problems I urge you to pay special attention to my suggestions about this in the final part of the book. For the time being I am going to describe a few easy exercises which will give strength and suppleness to your spinal muscles and hips. The hip flexors and extensors, stomach muscles as well as the back muscles all combine to protect and support the spine. Therefore if your weakness is in this area it is important for you to exercise each of these muscle groups. Use several blankets to lie on, or buy an exercise mat.

The Pelvic Tilt and Lift: TIME REQUIRED: 30 SECONDS. This exercise is absolutely essential if your lower back is under stress from standing for long periods in the one spot. Lie on the floor with your arms by your sides, knees bent so that your feet are flat on the floor. Pull your stomach in while flattening your spine against the floor so that there is no space between your lower back and the floor. Use your hand to check that this is so. If you can slide your hand in under your lower back you need to flatten more. Breathe slowly with each repetition. When you have mastered this movement lift the buttocks off the floor by contracting them and using your stomach muscles. Then lower by rolling gently down the vertebrae.

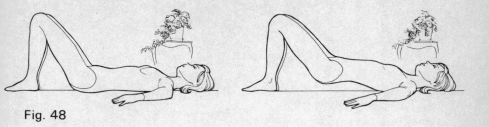

Fig. 48

The Lower Back Limber: TIME REQUIRED: 30 SECONDS. Lie on the floor in the same position as for the exercise above. Keeping your knees together and feet flat on the floor, swing your knees over from one side to the other. Try to keep your back stretched and flattened against the floor down the full length of the spine. Do this ten times.

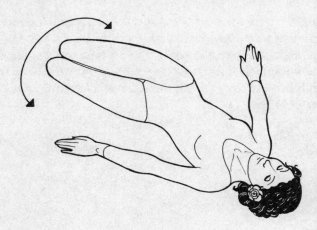

Fig. 49

The Spine Stretch and Relax: TIME REQUIRED: 1 MINUTE. Lie on your back and bring the knees up to your chest. Flatten your back. Put your arms around your knees and draw them as close to you as possible. Now bring up your head to meet the knees. Do this three times. Then in the same position cross your legs at the ankles and grasp each foot in your hands, keep your chin in and body completely relaxed. Rock backwards and forwards.

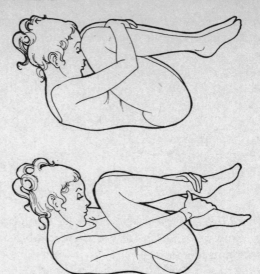

Fig. 50

Hip Limber: TIME REQUIRED: 60 SECONDS. This quick exercise will tone up muscles and improve the circulation. Lie on your back, flex the right foot by bending it towards you and slowly stretch your right leg, lengthening it as much as possible. Now draw up the right hip, as high as you can. Do the same on the left side. Repeat each movement six times.

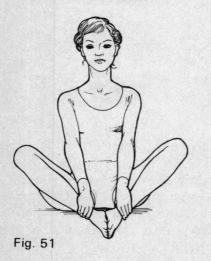

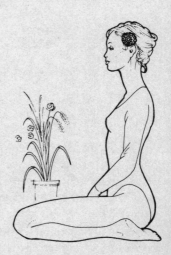

Fig. 51

Next rotate the right hip outwards as far as you can, then inwards. Repeat with the left hip and do the movements six times for each. A variation on these movements is to sit on the floor, tailor fashion. Sit with the soles of the feet touching and the knees turned out. Be sure to keep your back straight. This rotates the hips outwards. Sit in this position for a minute or so.

Next, kneel on the floor and sit between your heels. This movement rotates the hips inwards. If you cannot do this at first just go as far as you can. Build up gradually and do not strain the muscles. These exercises will keep the hip joints mobile and help prevent arthritic conditions from developing.

The Spine Aligner: TIME REQUIRED: 30 SECONDS. Stand against a wall with the knees bent and feet slightly turned out. Contract your stomach muscles as hard as you can, at the same time forcing the small of your back against the wall. You will find that the pelvis will naturally tilt upwards. Stretch your neck, keeping your chin parallel to the floor. Gradually straighten your knees. Hold this position for a slow count of ten. Keep your breathing normal. At first repeat the movements three times. Later you can work up to six repetitions if you wish. You should try to memorise this feeling of good posture and make it a habit.

The Cobra: TIME REQUIRED: 30 SECONDS. This is an easy yoga technique to master, but do not underestimate its effectiveness. Many of my clients tell me that it is one of the most helpful exercises I teach them. Lie face down on the floor. *Making sure your hips stay in contact with the ground*, push slowly upwards with your arms until the elbows

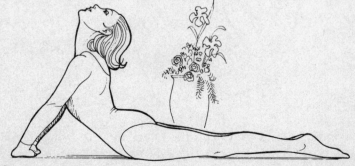

Fig. 52

are straight. Arch your back as far as you can, and allow your head to move back naturally with the push-up, as shown in Figure 52. Hold for a slow count of seven and repeat five times.

Stomach: TOTAL TIME REQUIRED: 90 SECONDS. Apart from the fact that a flat, smoothly muscled stomach is far more attractive than a paunch, there is a very sound health reason for making certain you maintain good muscle tone in this region of the body. Behind the protective abdominal wall lies not only the intricate digestive tract but also such vital organs as kidneys and liver. To function properly these must be well supported and held in the correct relationship to one another. Weak muscles, unable to perform these essential duties adequately, lead to the risk of *prolapse* in later life. In this condition the organs drop out of place and it may take major surgery to put things right again.

The Body Sense procedures will not restore years of neglect overnight, but they will gradually help to firm up the muscles so that you both look and feel in better shape. Even before you notice any change in appearance, however, they will have improved the circulation and so helped the muscles to grow and work more efficiently.

The Knees-Up/Sit-Up: There is no minimum time for this exercise as even one successful attempt is highly commendable at first. It should not normally take more than 6 seconds to complete however. Repeat several times gradually increasing the repetitions daily.

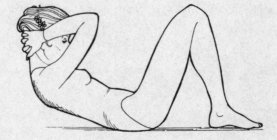

Fig. 53

Lie on your back and bend the knees so as to bring the heels as close as possible to your buttocks. The reason I suggest you adopt this position, rather than the more usual straight-legs posture for doing a sit up, is that it makes the stomach muscles, rather than the hip flexors, do most of the work. In addition, should you be suffering from any back trouble, using the knees-up position avoids the risk of strains.

To carry out the movement put your hands behind your head and attempt to sit up so that you can touch your elbows to your knees. Do not become discouraged if this proves impossible on the first few tries. Persevere and you will manage it in the end. Each attempt, even if unsuccessful, helps to strengthen the muscles and improve the blood flow.

The Double Leg Lift: TIME REQUIRED: 60 SECONDS. This is an easier technique than the one above, but it still works well to tone another set of stomach muscles and eliminate unsightly flabbiness.

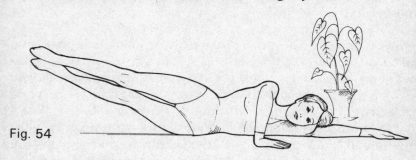

Fig. 54

Start by lying on your left side, your left hand extended above your head with the palm flat on the floor. Rest your head on the left arm and cross the right in front of your body. Keeping your ankles and knees straight together raise your legs off the floor as high as possible and then lower them again. Do not worry if you are unable to lift your legs very far at first. You will soon increase the strength in your stomach muscles, and so improve the height of the lift, if you practice this technique regularly. Do three repetitions on the left side then roll over and repeat exactly the same movements on your right side three more times. Later you can increase the number and height of raises to whatever time and comfort allows.

Wrists: Huen-Sau (Circling Hands). TIME REQUIRED: 60 SECONDS. This is a marvellous strengthening exercise derived from Chinese yoga which also gives remarkable suppleness to both wrist and forearm. It may be carried out while sitting or standing and you should perform three repetitions with each hand. As is so often the case with Oriental exercises the name Huen-Sau, or circling hands, provides a very good idea of what sort of movements to expect.

Start by extending your left arm straight out in front of you, palm upwards, thumb tucked in.

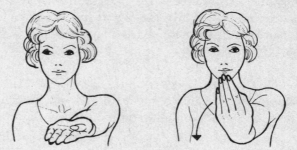

Fig. 55

Now bend the wrist so that you make a right angle of your hand and forearm. Keeping the elbow as still as you can, slowly rotate your hand in a clockwise direction. Turn it as far as possible *without* allowing your arm to twist at the elbow. You may find it easier to do this, at first, if you grasp the left elbow to keep it motionless. With a little practice, however, it will become quite easy to relax the wrist muscles and allow the hand to flop limply to the right. Do not become discouraged if, at first, you find it impossible to turn the wrist as far as I have shown in the drawing. Such suppleness can only be achieved after carrying out the exercise regularly for a week or so.

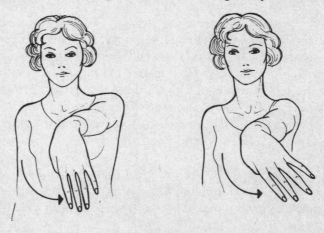

Fig. 56

When the hand has been turned as far as possible, hold this position for a couple of seconds, as in Figure 56. Close your hand very suddenly to make a fist. As you do so relax the muscles in your hand and arm. This is a movement which takes a little while to perfect, but the benefits are so great they make the effort well worthwhile. It is especially helpful if you play sports such as tennis or squash which make great demands on the wrists.

Return from the clenched fist position to the starting point and repeat the whole sequence twice more. Next turn your attention to the right wrist. You do exactly the same movements but this time rotate in an anti-clockwise direction so that the hand turns towards the left.

The key points of this exercise are:

*That the elbow keeps as still as possible.

*That the hand is allowed to rotate as far as possible. In time to the extent shown in the drawing.

*That you snap sharply into a clenched fist and simultaneously relax the muscles. I suggest that you practice before a mirror to ensure the hand is circling correctly. If this technique is being carried out correctly you will experience a considerable tension in the wrist and on the underside of the forearm. Do not be concerned about this. It merely shows that the muscles are being successfully loosened and strengthened.

Upper Leg: TOTAL TIME REQUIRED: 2 MINUTES 30 SECONDS.

The Ballet Bend and Reach: TIME REQUIRED: 60 SECONDS. Pain in the hamstrings of the upper leg, together with the stiffness and lack of agility which this uncomfortable problem involves, can best be prevented by using some of the movements which dancers employ when warming up their muscles.

Stand with your heels together and your toes just far enough apart so that you feel comfortable and balanced. Extend your right hand straight out to the side while keeping the left relaxed at your side.

Sweep your right hand down to touch the space between your feet. Use a wide, circular movement but do not worry if you are unable to touch the ground at first. When you feel the muscles at the back of the leg restricting you, hold the position for a moment. Concentrate on relaxing those muscles. You will then find that you can bend further forward. Never force.

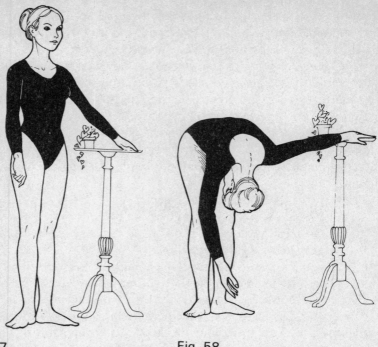

Fig. 57   Fig. 58

Now straighten up smoothly sweeping the right arm up in front of the body. As you do this your arm should be what dancers call 'rounded'. That is with the wrist and elbow curved so that the arm forms a perfect half-circle. Sweep the rounded arm up in front of you as you straighten and bring it over your head as shown in Figure 59.

Do not stop in this position but bend backwards a little, still holding your right arm above your head in the rounded position. This back bend movement is important because it counters any stress imposed on the back when bending forwards. By adding this touch to your upper leg movements you will also improve the back muscles. The rounded arm gives the rest of the body the optimal position for toning up the muscles and helps you move smoothly.

You might like to complete this exercise by one further movement which is a general muscle toner for the waist. From the straight standing posture, with your curved right arm still over your head pull your body upwards and bend to the left side. Allow the weight

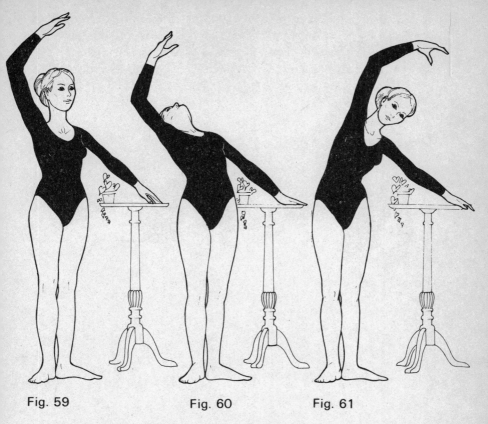

Fig. 59   Fig. 60   Fig. 61

of the curved arm to help draw you to the left. Make sure your left
shoulder stays in position and does not move backwards.

After this, return to the standing straight position, drop your right
arm to your side and relax it. Repeat the procedure for the left side of
the body by bringing up the left arm over the head in the rounded
position and finally bending to the *right* side. Repeat the whole
sequence 3 times.

Jazz Dancer's Leg Swing: TIME REQUIRED: 60 SECONDS. Here is
another excellent upper leg exercise that you can use in conjunction
with, or as an alternative to, the ballet bend and reach. Once again it
is taken from the dance, this time the world of jazz. It is very good for
toning and limbering the thigh muscles.

Hold onto a chair with your left hand. Stand with the feet turned out just enough to feel comfortably balanced. Keeping the weight on your foot swing your right leg to the right side as shown by the arrows. Make sure your right knee and toes are pointing to the side as in the illustration below. The working leg should be slightly bent. The supporting leg straight.

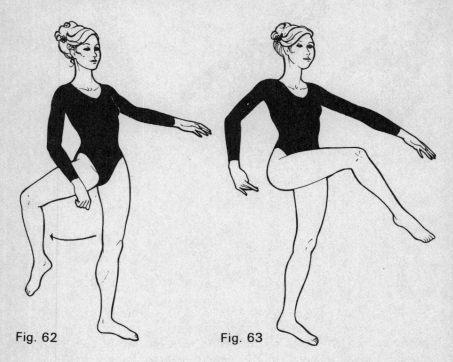

Fig. 62   Fig. 63

Now, *immediately* swing the right leg back in front of the body. If you want to make the movement as much like that of a professional jazz dancer as possible – and this is the most effective way of carrying out the technique – you should brush the ground with your foot with each swing of the right leg. As it touches the ground the foot should, for a moment, return to the starting position: that is slightly turned outwards.

Finally, swing your right leg back to the right, again brushing the floor on the way. The important points to remember for this technique to be effective are:

* Bend the working knee slightly. Keep the supporting knee straight.

* Keep the toes pointed.
* Brush the ground lightly.

Do ten repetitions of this movement with each leg. As the thighs get back into shape you can increase the number to as many as time and comfort permit.

The Demiplié: TIME REQUIRED: 90 SECONDS. The demiplié is a movement so basic to ballet that no routine could be performed without it. There is no need to have had any dance training to use this exercise, however, and its benefits are considerable whatever type of movement you want to carry out.

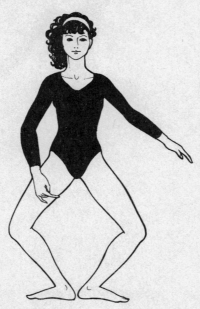

Fig. 64

Stand with your heels together and the toes turned out. The ideal angle is about 90°, but you should adopt the one which feels most comfortable. Use a chair or table to help your balance as you do this exercise.

Keeping your weight over your little toes, as far as you can, bend at the knees and come slowly down with your heels flat on the ground. This is essential if the movement is to be carried out correctly. Your backside should be tucked well in so that the base of the spine points straight down to the floor.

When you are down as far as you can manage, come back up to your starting position. Now rise up onto the balls of your feet. Keep your stomach flat and pull up your ribcage.

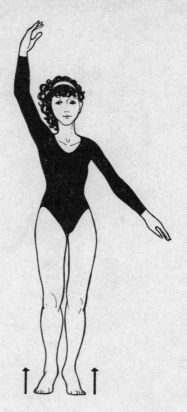

Fig. 65

Now lower your heels gently, at the same time drawing up the rest of your body. As you sink you must apply an equal and opposite upward effort against the ribcage. When done correctly this will give the feeling of being caught between two opposing forces, the one drawing you downwards the other pulling you upwards. It may take a little practice to achieve this sensation, but you will know right away when the movement is being done successfully. The feeling is delightful and gives you a tremendous sense of lightness.

Knee: Full Plié. TIME REQUIRED: 30 SECONDS. As with the other techniques I have described for bringing strength and suppleness to the legs, this exercise is a method used by dancers to give them the endurance and agility on which their success depends. It will ensure that you can move easily and gracefully too.

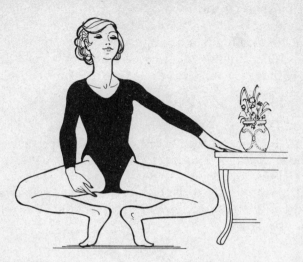

Fig. 66

Stand with your heels together and your toes turned out as much as you can up to an angle of 90°. Support yourself by resting one hand on a table or chair. Now, keeping your back straight and weight on the little toes, slowly bend at the knees. Continue to lower your body, the back held straight, until your heels lift from the floor. Resist the tendency for the heels to rise, so that your body has been lowered as fully as possible before this happens. The lifting of the ankles is a signal for you to start straightening up. Do this slowly and gracefully. As you come up try to get your heels flat on the floor again as quickly as you can.

The action of the heels is important to this technique because the muscles involved in heel action have a beneficial effect on the knees while also strengthening the achilles tendons. Now rise up on to the balls of the feet. Lower the heels while pulling the body upwards from the waist so that you get a lovely two way stretch.

Lower Legs: Ankles. Strong, supple ankles are essential to muscle health because it is impossible to move naturally or hold oneself correctly unless they are in good shape. The total time needed for these exercises is two minutes.

Ankle Exercise: Stand up straight and rest your hand on a chair or other waist high object. Start by pointing your foot straight out in front, knees straight with the toe touching the ground. Now flex your foot, raising it towards you. Then turn your foot inwards from the ankle and hold it for a slow count of seven. Next, return to the starting position. Finally, flex your foot again and turn it outwards from the ankle, holding for a slow count of seven. Repeat this sequence with the other foot and relax the feet afterwards by shaking them one at a time.

Zenkutsu Dachi: TIME REQUIRED: 60 SECONDS. The next technique is taken from the Kabuki, the ritual Japanese theatre. One of its many formalised stances, the Zenkutsu Dachi is often used by performers miming fighting sequences. When combined with a bouncing motion, I have found it to be one of the best possible methods of improving and strengthening muscle tone in the ankles, and stretching the calves.

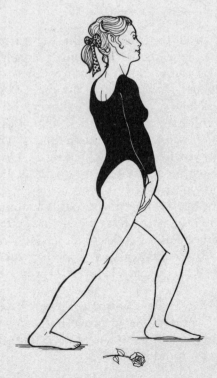

Fig. 67

Stand upright, bend your left knee and extend your right leg behind you keeping the arms relaxed at your sides. By adopting this stance you will have reduced your height some six inches.

Make a series of small, bouncing movements by raising and lowering your right heel. Remember to keep the right leg straight during this movement. After a dozen bounces change to the right leg.

This is a marvellous exercise for warming your muscles before playing any sport, especially those such as golf, tennis or squash which demand supple ankles. To complete your ankle exercises sit in a comfortable chair, stretch out one leg and point the toe as firmly as you can. Then flex the foot by bending it upwards. Do this half a dozen times and finish by rotating the ankle for ten seconds. Change over legs and repeat.

This brings us to the end of the pain prevention exercises. Create a programme to suit your individual needs and start using it right away. As you do so, continue to read this book and introduce any other exercises which are appropriate to your current health situation. In Part Four I will be looking at ways of helping your body combat the stresses and strains of everyday living which can take such a powerful toll of your emotional well-being.

PART FOUR

The Body Sense way to peace of mind

Modern life is not merely extremely stressful, it has also produced a far greater awareness of the harmful effects of such stress. Doctors warn constantly of the threats posed by hypertension; articles in the press alert us to the dangers of becoming too tense; there are TV programmes describing the consequences of constant pressure at work and in the home. The result is that people not only suffer from stresses arising from the way they live, but make matters worse by getting stressed over the risks they run by being stressed! It often looks like the ultimate vicious circle. The ever spreading infection of anxiety, depression and worry. 'I smoke to help keep me calm when I think about the dangers of smoking,' said one of my clients. But behind his quip was a considerable truth. We are constantly exposed to situations which can undermine our psychological resistance and so make us increasingly vulnerable to both mental and physical sickness. No wonder that the manufacture of tranquillisers is now a billion dollar industry!

How to survive? Some people try to excape stress by a change of lifestyle. They give up the pressures of business life and seek sanctuary in a quiet country cottage. Sometimes it works. Often they find that one type of stress has merely been replaced by another. They may for example have exchanged too much daily stimulation for too little. Others may try to cope by damping down their nervous systems by the use of drink or drugs.

Body Sense Therapy offers you an approach which is far better since it does not attempt to change your bodily responses by means of medication or your lifestyle through a drastic change in direction. Rather it offers a method of coping with stress by giving your body a chance to build new and better defences for dealing effectively with everyday strains and tensions. The aim is to enjoy the stimulation which stress can provide while preventing it from creating emotional and physical havoc. In this part of the book I am going to tell you how that desirable goal can be achieved.

Why stress sours your system

Most people know what it means to feel anxious. The sudden panic before an important interview or crucial test is familiar to almost everybody. If you recall such a moment of psychological distress, perhaps a time when you had to defend yourself in an angry scene, present arguments in the face of stiff opposition, or give a talk to a large group of people, the way you felt will come flooding back. You probably found yourself breathing more rapidly, your heart began to thump wildly, you may have started to sweat profusely, to tremble or feel faint. At the same moment it is likely there were uncomfortable mental changes as well, confusion and failures of memory, an inability to concentrate or follow the thread of an argument.

All these are the obvious consequences of excessive stress. Much less well known, however, are more subtle and less easily detected changes which occur inside the body. For example, there is a redirection of the circulation so that more blood reaches the brain and limbs while less is supplied to the digestive system. There are changes in digestion as well, which is why anxiety so frequently makes you feel physically sick. As stress increases the muscles become more tense. The greater the stress the greater this tension. This dulls the sixth sense, putting you further out of touch with your body, and causes the muscles to function much less efficiently in their role of energy storehouse and regulator of the body's chemistry.

When tension due to constant stress becomes a habit, it influences not only the way you feel but also the way you look. Frequent tenseness causes the muscles involved to lose their tone and become inelastic, setting the body into a particular expression or posture rather like clay hardening in a mould. The facial muscles reflect internal strain by developing wrinkles and folds, by sagging unattractively and appearing prematurely old. Constriction of the small blood vessels near the surface of the skin harms the complexion by starving the cells which also become clogged with self-produced poisons. A healthy glow is rapidly replaced by an unhealthy pallor that is such a marked feature of somebody suffering from uncontrolled stress.

More people visit the dermatologist because of stress than for any other reason. Stress actually *causes* some skin conditions, while aggravating others and there now seems to be a link between stress and allergies. I have noticed too with many of my clients that they develop vesicles – tiny bubbles of colourless fluid on their fingers or feet, also pink patches or 'allergic' skin reactions only when they are facing traumatic periods in their life.

When we have grown used to excessive tension in our everyday lives it can become such a familiar companion that we no longer take any notice of it. It is like somebody living next to a railway line being undisturbed by the trains after a few weeks. But we cannot go on ignoring it in quite the same way as those trains. In the end there will be a day of reckoning when our health simply breaks under the unacceptable strain.

So the first step in using Body Sense to survive stress is to find out just how much tension you are currently enduring and what, if anything, this situation is doing to your health. You can do this by means of the short questionnaire below. Simply tick those statements which apply to your present lifestyle and then add up the number of ticks.

Stress check

1: My sleep is often disturbed by ideas circling madly through my brain. ✓

2: I find that small things easily irritate me. ✓

3: I am usually in a rush to get somewhere or do something.

4: In my dreams I am frequently the victim of a situation which has got out of control. ✓

5: I find myself feeling anxious for no apparent reason. ✓

6: I find it hard to eat my meals slowly. ✓

7: I regularly experience one of the following (a) shortness of breath (b) trembling hands (c) sweating palms (d) rapidly beating heart. ✓

8: I spend a lot of my time worrying about what is going to happen to me. ✓

9: When climbing a flight of stairs I usually take them two at a time.

10: These days I often think life is getting on top of me. ✓
11: I frequently wake in the early hours and cannot get back to sleep. ✓
12: After work is finished I find it very hard to sit down and relax. ✓

What your answers tell you

If you found that no more than *one* of the twelve statements applied to you, you are coping well. Keep an eye on events, however, to make sure your psychological health continues in this satisfactory condition.

A score of between two and three suggests that although stress is not yet likely to prove a threat you must be careful not to allow matters to get out of control. I suggest you use the first set of Body Sense techniques described below to help contain the situation.

If you answered 'yes' to four or more statements, then there is a distinct possibility that excessive levels of stress are undermining your health. It is time to take appropriate preventive measures and you should make use of all the techniques contained in this part of the book.

Let us begin by looking at some of the psychological procedures that are helpful in relieving damagingly high stress levels. I will then tell you how various movement and massage techniques can be used in order to ease away the physical tensions produced by excessive anxiety or depression.

Thought stopping

This technique can be used anywhere and at any time to prevent the relentless flow of ideas which are making you feel worried, unhappy or upset. Although it sounds amazingly simple, the procedure has been shown to be one of the most powerful mental weapons yet devised for destroying all those counter-productive concerns that can dominate our thoughts at times of excessive stress.

As tension begins to build up, and unhelpful notions start circulating through the mind, all you have to do to call a halt is say, very firmly: STOP! Then immediately start to remember a favourite tune. As you do so, allow your body to go as limp as a rag doll. When imagining the music make certain you play it through note by note in your mind. After only a few bars you will detect a considerable reduction in physical tension as the distracting worries are driven from the centre of the mental stage. If you want to use the technique with other people about then it is OK to tell your thoughts to STOP either under your breath or silently. But it is essential to make the command incisive. It should be the kind of sharp, urgent order you would give to a small child about to knock a priceless vase to the ground!

Mind travel

Here is a method for fighting stress by using your mind to relax both itself and the body through the use of mental imagery. You can do it while sitting, lying or even – with a little practice – when walking around. Developed by American fitness expert Dr Art Ulene it utilises mental imagery to inwind tensions and drive away worries.

While learning how to use Mind Travel you should sit or lie comfortably in a quiet room, close your eyes and breathe slowly and deeply for about fifteen seconds. Now imagine, as vividly as possible that you are in a very relaxing spot, perhaps a sun filled glade in the woods or on a quiet beach. Involve all your senses in this fantasy scene so that you can almost smell the soft aroma of the trees and grass, or the salty tang of the oceans. Feel the sun warm on your body; hear the rustle of leaves or waves breaking gently on the shore while 'seeing' every detail of your surroundings.

Observe this tranquil setting at your leisure until some living creature appears. The first one to pop into your imagination will do. Dr Ulene's special animal is a rabbit called Corky! I want you to imagine yourself approaching this animal, who is quite without fear, and calling him towards you. Get to know him. Ask questions, such as his name, where he comes from, what he likes to eat and so on. You will be amazed to find your brain automatically provides the answers! When you are familiar with the animal start explaining your problems to him. Completely unburden yourself by telling him everything that is worrying you. Do not hold back anything. When you have finished, bid the animal goodbye and say you will return. Then, slowly, open your eyes and return to the real world.

Perhaps this technique sounds rather foolish at first reading. Some of my clients have laughed aloud when I suggested they use it.

But amusement invariably turned to astonishment and relief after only a few sessions. Astonishment that an animal really *did* appear on the scene, and they *could* find out every detail they wanted about him. Relief that they had at last found an intensely private but totally effective method for sorting out their problems. It is truly remarkable just how powerful this mental imagery usually proves. You really do feel that your worries have been brought into perspective simply by sharing them, silently but frankly, with your fantasy animal friend.

How can it work so effectively? There is nothing magical about the technique which is founded in sound psychological theory. Because you involve all your five senses when creating the original scene you turn your attention inwards and so prevent yourself from focusing on worries in the outside world. Because you are trying to construct a complicated mental image, your mind is unable to concentrate on the anxiety producing problems and gradually enters a state of relaxed detachment in which the unconscious comes to exert a more powerful influence than was previously possible.

Each time you enter this fantasy kingdom it is important to conjure up the same creature so that he quickly becomes an old and trusted 'friend'. When this happens, and it usually takes only a few sessions of mind travel for the 'friendship' to flourish, the mental image becomes linked with a feeling of relaxation and the release from everyday problems. In time you will find that there is no need to develop the scene in all its earlier details. Just by picturing your special 'friend' a sensation of peace floods the body and mind, easing away physical and psychological tensions.

The Zen stress releaser

Finally here is a psychological procedure taken from the ancient art of Zen which my clients find works marvellously any time they need to reduce stress symptoms quickly. Simply sit quietly with your back straight and start to breathe gently. Become aware of *all* the sensations around you as vividly as possible. Take in the sights and sounds, the smells, the feel of your body and the very air you inhale. As you breathe in try to imagine that all these multitudinous sensations are being sucked into your body. As you breathe out relax your muscles and this time attempt to let your mind go completely blank, as though the exhalation of air had silenced all sensation. Repeat as often as you like for five or ten minutes. You will find it works wonders for jangled nerves and a tense body.

A massage relaxer

I am going to start by looking at a rapid self massage technique that can ease tension and stress from the muscles and so help soothe the mind. Use it any time anxiety strikes.

The first indications that you are becoming anxious include a dry mouth, an uncomfortable feeling in the stomach and a rapid heart. Stretch as hard as you can right from your toes to your fingertips. This puts your body into a condition where relaxation can occur more readily. Pay particular attention to areas where tension seems to accumulate most easily – the hands and feet, neck and shoulders, the tongue, jaw and forehead. Feel warmth enveloping your whole body. Breathe slowly and deeply from the abdomen. If possible gaze at some relaxing sight, such as a tree or a flower. Now begin the massage as follows:

One:
Grasp the shoulder muscles on one side of the neck pulling them up with the fingers and palm of the opposite hand. Hold 30 seconds. Repeat in the middle of the shoulder and also at the end. This will ease a lot of the tension in that muscle. Make sure hand and arm hang down relaxed.

Two:
Now move your hand to grasp your shoulder muscle directly in the centre. Carry out a series of rapid small shrugging movements and finish off by rotating the shoulder backward. Remember to maintain a gentle but firm grasp of the shoulder muscle throughout.

Three:
Stroke down from the base of the skull to the shoulders with the fingers, using fairly firm pressure.

Four:
Place your hand at the back of the neck and knead it between the

fingers and the palm of the hand as though you were picking up a kitten by the scruff of the neck. Move the muscles from side to side.

Five:

Still grasping the muscle in the back of the neck, move your head up and down, as if nodding. Then move it from side to side as if signalling 'no'. Finish by drawing circles with your nose in the air. Repeat each of these movements about a dozen times, remembering to relax your head, jaw, face throughout – but don't let go of the neck with your hand.

Six:

Do deep friction massage 1" each side of the 7th cervical vertebra (that prominent bone at the base of the neck sometimes known as the dowager's hump) to the base of the skull. Now work all along the base of the skull, round the ears and into the scalp.

Take a warm (not too hot) bath to which you've added some essential oils (see page 61) known especially for their calming and soothing effect on the nerves. Add a few drops of any or a mixture of the following: jasmin, benzoin, lavender, marjoram or neroli (orange blossom). Once you have mastered these techniques you will be well on the way to halting all the mild thoughts that spoil your concentration, undermine your happiness and prevent you from enjoying restful sleep. To ease away bodily tensions even more deeply I suggest you use a quick movement exercise. This takes only one minute to carry out, and my clients find it especially beneficial.

The swing-release

Stand with your legs slightly further apart than the shoulder width, toes pointing outwards. Bend forward at the waist and let your head and arms hang down. Relax so that hands, arms and head flop in space like a puppet with broken strings.

Now I want you to shake your arms and hands as if they were rags. Waggle them as limply as you like for fifteen seconds. Then relax again. After a few moments begin to swing your body slowly from side to side, remembering to remain as relaxed as possible. Continue to do this for half a minute and then relax once more.

Straighten up slowly, from the waist, leaving your head and arms dangling limply as you do so. At the end of this short exercise you should feel refreshed, alert and able to cope with life more easily.

Regard all these rapid techniques, both psychological and physical, as your first line of defence against excessive stress. You can master them with a minimum of difficulty, use them in a matter of minutes, and enjoy the relief they provide wherever and whenever the need arises.

How to pick yourself up when life puts you down

My clients often ask me whether there is any Body Sense technique which could help to boost morale when the going gets rough. Some natural means for picking you up when life threatens to drag you down, after a bad day at work, for example, or when you have received upsetting news, following a disheartening set-back or at moments when the world looks black.

The method I usually suggest is a sort of psychological pep-pill – which turns on the resources of the body rather than relying on the effects of any drug. It was created centuries ago by monks in China's famous Shao Lin monastery to relieve the harshness of their spartan lives and make their minds more receptive to philosophical thoughts. You can use it just as successfully to revitalise your whole system.

You should open a window and stay close by it so that you can draw fresh air into your lungs as you carry out the sequence of movements I shall describe.

Stand with your feet together, hands turned inwards and finger-tips touching, elbows held in front of the body.

Inhale slowly and very deeply through your nose. As you breathe in I want you to start rising up onto your toes while simultaneously raising your hands. All three actions must take place together.

The timing must be such that, at the moment your lungs are so full of air you can no longer draw a breath, you are standing on tiptoe with your hands approximately level with the midline of the chest. Hold this position for about two seconds.

Turn your palms downwards and push your hands slowly towards the ground, sinking back on your heels and exhaling slowly as you do so. Here again all three movements must occur together and your timing must be adjusted so that you have expelled the last gasp of air

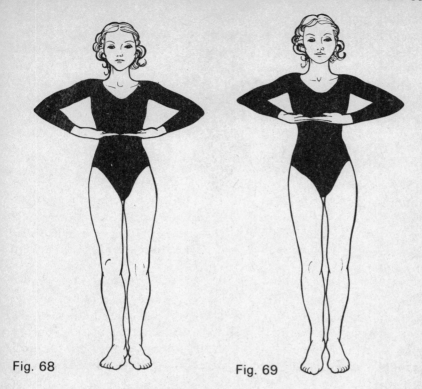

Fig. 68   Fig. 69

from your lungs, and placed your feet flat on the ground once more, with your hands returned to the starting position, all at the same moment. As you breathe out you should produce an audible 'haaaaaaaaaah' sound.

The method of breathing is important. You must keep the ribcage flat throughout the exercise. Do not expand or contract the chest at all when inhaling and exhaling. Instead suck air in and force it out again by the actions of your abdominal muscles. My clients often find that, at first, this type of breathing comes more easily if they imagine a large balloon inside their stomach which is inflated when they inhale and deflated as they breathe out again. As your hands move upwards try to feel that they are drawing air into your body and down into the balloon. As you bring them down again imagine their effect as pushing the air out again. Repeat the movement ten times.

If you perform this exercise properly you will quickly feel a

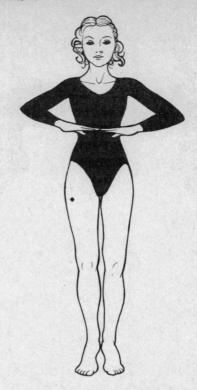

Fig. 70

delightful sensation of relaxed and elated detachment. If you had been irritable, frustrated, depressed or unhappy earlier these negative and distressing moods ought to be considerably diminished. You should be more confident about your ability to cope, see the really important issues before you more clearly and be in a far better shape to cope with life's demands. It is a heady feeling that persists for between fifteen minutes and an hour. After which, if you need another quick 'pick-me-up' you need only carry out the exercise again.

The next technique I want to tell you about also comes from China and is called Yeun Chun or Eternal Springtime. Although slightly more complicated to perform than the Shao Lin technique its effects are more profound and longer lasting. The movements you are going to learn were invented by Hua T'o, a famous physician of the Tang dynasty who based them on the animals and birds which he observed during long years of meditation in the wilderness. You will see this love of nature reflected in the distinctly animal-like actions involved: the slithering of a snake, the graceful swinging of the crane's neck, the flashing motion of a fish in the clear water. Hua T'o believed that the unrestricted movements which he saw in wild creatures were far more health enhancing than the restrained, awkward and inhibited ones men so often adopted. Hua T'o and the disciples who came to use and teach his methods, saw the movements he devised as a means of improving muscle efficiency and inducing a feeling of deep relaxation. If you follow my instructions carefully you too should discover the state of blissful tranquillity which so impressed those early Chinese enthusiasts. It is a feeling of being both relaxed and yet alert, soothed but at the same time stimulated. If you have difficulty in sleeping, or wake up in the morning still feeling tired, then perform Yeun Chun just before going to bed. You should find that everyday worries slip effortlessly from your shoulders so that you can enjoy rapid and restful sleep.

Incidently, the title Eternal Springtime was bestowed by Hua T'o's grateful followers, many of whom lived for more than a century but remained mentally and physically vigorous throughout their lives.

The most essential thing to remember is that to be successful all the movements in Yeun Chun must be performed *very, very slowly*. Some, indeed, have to be carried out so slowly that it might not appear to an observer that you were actually moving at all! While doing each one, it is also important to focus your entire mind on the part of the body involved, and to move smoothly, easily and effortlessly. You must avoid any suggestion of abruptness or jerkiness in your actions.

In order to explain what you must do in the clearest manner, I have separated the various movements, numbering and describing each one in turn. But, when carrying them out, each should be allowed to flow into the next without any pause or hesitation. The best way to achieve this is to read the descriptions in turn and study the illustration. Then practise carrying out one particular part of the technique a few times before moving on to the next one. You might find it helpful, if you have a cassette recorder, to make a tape of the instructions. Once you have mastered each of them to your satisfaction run through the whole sequence. None of them is difficult and my clients usually find they can learn the entire sequence after no more than half a dozen sessions.

When carrying out the movements remain relaxed at all times. Exert only sufficient muscular effort to perform the action required. The parts of the body which are not being used should be kept as free from tension as you can manage.

Before starting loosen any tight clothing and remove your shoes. Now begin as follows:

One:

Stand with arms at your side, palms facing towards the rear, feet about as far apart as your shoulders with the toes pointing to the front and your knees slightly bent. Rise slowly on your toes and

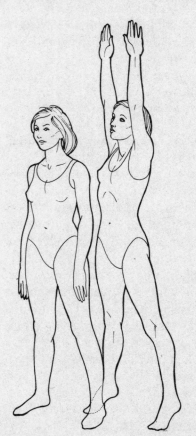

Fig. 71

simultaneously lift your arms directly to the front keeping the elbows and fingers straight. You should reach tiptoe at the moment your arms reach the vertical position shown in the illustration.

When your arms are fully raised above your head, the palms should be facing forward. The movement must take *at least* 10 seconds to complete. Because the tempo of each action is so important to its success, I would like you to practise completing this initial movement in not less than 10 seconds, so as to get a feeling for the correct speed. This is important because, unless I tell you otherwise, all the moves in Yuen Chun will be carried out at this tempo.

Two:

Moving at the same speed lower your arms sideways until they are parallel to the ground, palms facing downwards. At the same time sink back to the floor in such a way that the heels are flat as your arms reach the horizontal position.

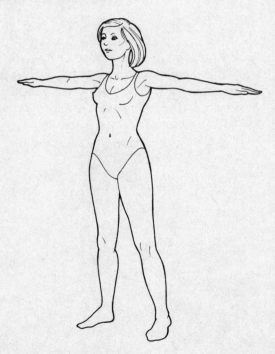

Fig. 72

Three:

Still moving at the same slow tempo, and keeping your arms stretched out to the side, bend your elbows to your sides until they are touching the body and turn the palms outwards.

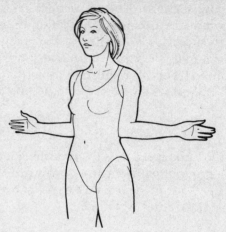

Fig. 73

Four:

With the elbows tucked in to your sides, bring your hands slowly towards one another keeping your arms parallel to the ground. As they come towards the front, bend your wrists gently backwards as if you were performing the movement in a pool and the water resistance was causing them to move out.

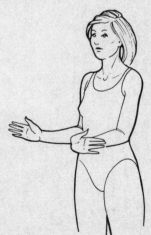

Fig. 74

Five:

Place the heel of your left hand over your right wrist, bending the left hand upwards so that the fingers point towards the ceiling as if in greeting. At the same time the right hand must bend inwards towards its own wrist with the fingers cupped. Both hands should be about 6–8 inches directly in front of the body at this point in the sequence.

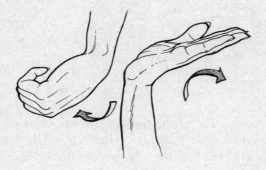

Fig. 75

Six:

This is the point at which I want you to really *slow down*! Start to move your left hand towards and your right away from its body. Do it in such a way that the motion is *barely perceptible*. Your left hand must reach a position about one inch in front of the body at the same moment the right hand arrives in a position with the arm almost fully extended. Practise so that both these moves are made together. When you perform this move your hands will, in fact, only be travelling a few inches. Yet I want you to do this action so gradually that it takes at least 12 seconds to carry out. Any faster and you are doing it too quickly. Using the counting method to give you the tempo when learning the movement.

Seven:

Without moving your arms, simply reverse the positions of the hands so that the fingers of the *right* hand are pointing upwards and the fingers of the left hand are curled inwards towards the wrist.

Eight:

Still moving as slowly as you possibly can, bring your right hand straight in towards your body and move your left straight away from the body. If this is carried out correctly your hands will meet about six inches in front of you. At this point keep moving them inwards and outwards until they reach the position shown in Figure 76.

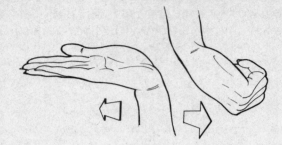

Fig. 76

Nine:

Do not move your arms, but reverse the position of the hands again so that the outstretched left hand is tilted up and the retracted right hand curls in to the wrist. Now start the superslow movements of your arms again, bringing the hands towards one another, passing the right over the left, so that the left hand is close to the body with the right arm fully extended.

Ten:

Right hand comes towards the body, left hand moves away. This is the start of a repeat of movements *six* to *nine* with the hand position reversed. As before do everything VERY SLOWLY.

Eleven:

Reverse position of hands.

Twelve

Left hand moves straight towards the body while your right hand away.

Thirteen:

Now reverse the position of your hands. Right tilted up, left curled.

Remember when carrying out all these movements your hands should barely seem to be moving at all. Look straight ahead, but focus all your attention on what your hands are doing. Try to clear your mind of any other thoughts. This may be difficult to achieve during the first few sessions, but it will come with practice. The harder it is to attain the mental focus and physical constraint demanded by Yuen Chun the more your mind and body are in need of its healing potency. By carrying out the Eternal Spring exercise regularly you will be able to banish the three 'Imps' that make tension free existence impossible: Impatience, Impulsiveness and Impetuousness. Only by expelling these destructive goblins from your lifestyle can you hope to achieve a health giving state of relaxation.

After a few sessions of the extra slow movements you will feel a tingling sensation in your arms. That is a sign that the circulation is starting to increase and that you are performing the movements correctly.

Fourteen:

Now we return to movements carried out at the 10 second speed. Straighten your fingers, and move your hands straight back to your sides allowing the forearms to brush your sides as you do so. Complete the movement with the palms turned towards the ceiling.

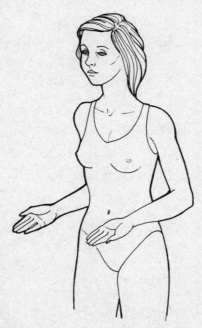

Fig. 77

Fifteen:

Move your feet slightly further apart. Then, keeping the right leg completely straight, bend your left knee as much as you can. As you come slowly down, twist your hips and shoulders in a clockwise direction and transfer almost all your weight to the left knee. Remain looking to the front, do not be tempted to turn your head as you rotate your hips and shoulders. Nose and toes must continue to point in the same direction.

Sixteen:

Extend your left arm straight out before you. As with all the movements in Yeun Chun do this slowly and smoothly. Form your left hand into the position shown in Figure 78 and, without bending the elbow, make a large sweeping circle with your arm (Figure 79).

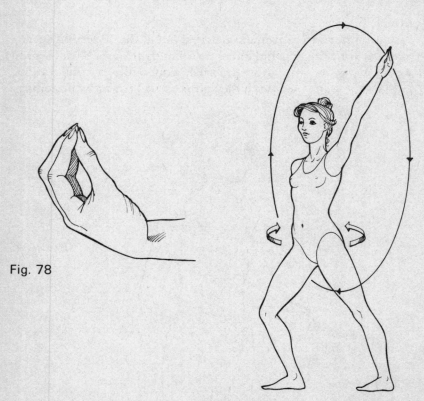

Fig. 78

Fig. 79

Seventeen:

Slowly straighten your left knee and bend the right, turning shoulders and hips in an anticlockwise direction, feet pointing forwards.

Eighteen:

Form the fingers of the right hand into the same shape as you did with the left a moment ago and make the same sweeping gesture, this time using the right arm.

Nineteen:

Turn shoulders and hips slowly towards the front, bring your hands back to your sides, palms turned outwards and fingers extended.

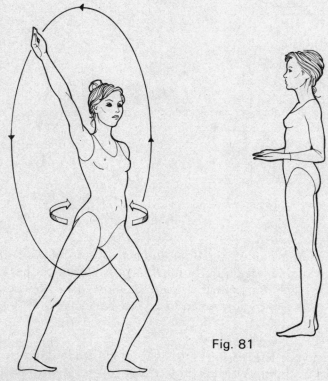

Fig. 81

Fig. 80

Twenty:

Raise your left leg, bending it at the knee so that your thigh comes as close as possible to the chest. You must stand on one leg for this movement and the next which may cause a balance problem at first. But it comes quickly with a little practice.

Twenty-one:

Lower your left leg slowly extending it out to the left.

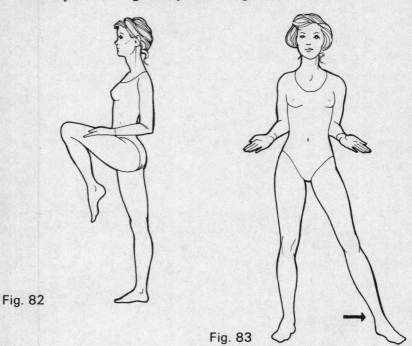

Fig. 82

Fig. 83

Twenty-two:

Swing the left leg up off the floor and across in front of the right leg. The toes should be pointed as much as possible and the left knee bent at a 45° angle. Remember to keep the movement slow and do not worry if, at first, you tend to lose your balance.

Twenty-three:

Straighten your left leg, keeping the toes pointed and return it to the starting position. You are now ready to repeat the last four movements, this time extending and using the right leg.

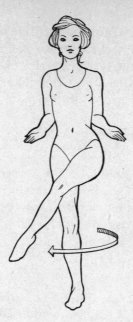

Fig. 84

Twenty-four

With the right leg exercise completed you are back in the position you were at the start of the leg movements. Continue by moving your arms slowly forward, angling them in towards the stomach and forming your fingers into the Tiger Claw.

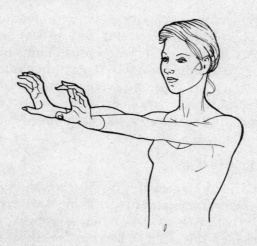

Fig. 85

Twenty-five:

This is the only movement in Yuen Chun which puts a part of the body under tension. As you slowly move your arms outwards and form the Tiger Claw, tense them as much as possible. If this is done properly they will start to shake slightly as if supporting a heavy load. Pretend that you are pushing as hard as you can against an invisible wall.

Twenty-six:

Open your hands and point the fingers straight out. Slowly bring the palms back towards the body, directing each palm towards the opposite shoulder. This movement, when performed correctly, will cause the forearms to cross one another about 8–10 inches in front of the body.

Twenty-seven:

Keeping the upper arms quite still, slowly move the forearms down to your sides. This will bring you back to the starting point. Now repeat the whole sequence again.

Like some of the other movements I describe in this book, Yuen Chun is far more time consuming to read about than it actually does to do! Indeed the whole sequence of movements, performed with the extreme slowness which I have emphasised throughout, takes only 5 minutes.

I have already described many benefits to mental and physical health which you will derive by using this ancient sequence of movements as part of your regular fitness programme. But the only way you are going to be truly convinced is not through any words of mine but from your own experience. So I do urge you to start practising Yuen Chun right away. Persevere for a week or so, carrying out two full sets of movements each day.

Soothing away your stresses

So far I have mainly discussed ways of relieving psychological tension. But it is just as important to ease bodily tensions as well, by soothing muscles which have grown taut through exposure to excessive stress. Unless this is done, their health is undermined, they are unable to work efficiently and your body is more vulnerable to aches and ailments.

You can safeguard yourself with a five minute massage session carried out after a particularly stressful day, or at any time when you feel under greater pressure than normal. The best time is following a relaxing bath, before you go to bed. But it can prove just as effective any time when you need to unwind quickly and completely. Use an aromatic oil of your choice.

Spine soothe

Let your head fall forward and place the fingertips of either hand on the part of the back where it merges with the neck. Here you will feel a protruding bone. This is the seventh cervical vertebra, the focal point for an extensive network of nerves in the back, neck and head.

Using your index and middle fingers, slowly circle around this bone applying moderate pressure. Repeat this about twenty times.

Neck soothe

Place the first and second fingers of each hand either side of the bony protrusion that indicates the seventh cervical vertebra. At each side of the spine is a slight depression, leading up towards the skull,

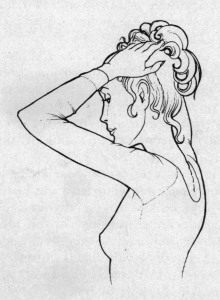

Fig. 86

which corresponds to the main tendons controlling head movements. It is here that stress and tension can exert much of their harmful effects. Carry out a deep friction massage, as described on page 65 while moving slowly up the neck until you reach the base of the skull.

Scalp and brow soothe

Without altering your head position place the fingertips of each hand on the temples. Using a gentle pressure slide your hands upwards towards the crown, lifting the scalp as you do so. When the heels of the hands are level with the tops of your ears, the fingers will no longer be in contact with the scalp, but you should continue by pressing the hands against the scalp and pushing it upwards, as shown in figure 86. Repeat six times.

Now straighten your head. Place the thumb pads on top of each eye-socket, just beneath the eye-brows. Exert gentle pressure. Lift and stroke slowly outwards until you reach the temples. Next place the thumb pads on the eyebrows, lift and stroke outwards once more. Move them just above the eyebrows and repeat the lifting and stroking motion. The procedure is to continue to move your hands in this way, about half an inch at a time, until the hairline is reached. Repeat the entire sequence twice more. Finish off by doing deep friction all over the scalp with the finger tips.

Stomach soothe

When you are anxious and upset all your tension accumulates in the stomach area. Just place your hands on a baby's stomach when he is crying and he will respond by relaxing. Rub or press gently your cat or dog's stomach when he is lying on his back, see how he relaxes even more. Buddhist monks meditate by breathing into the stomach and 'massaging' the area in a circle 50 times.

Lie down and bend up your knees. Place your right hand on your stomach, just below the navel, and your left hand just above the navel. Circle your hands clockwise slowly and rhythmically, while at the same time applying moderate pressure. Do this for about 15 seconds and then cross over your hands so they touch opposite sides of the body. Press firmly and draw your hands together, gradually reducing the pressure so that, by the time they meet, your fingers are merely stroking the skin. Do this six times.

Now, with very loose and relaxed hands gently squeeze the abdomen, up and down. Gently rock the abdomen from side to side using the fingertips and the heel of the hand. Next place one hand on top of the other and do a short series of gentle vibrations. Then repeat on the muscles along the side, cupping the muscles in your hands and lifting them as you exhale, four times. This will also help to relieve tension in your lower back as well.

Lower back soothe

Place your hands on your hips with thumbs touching the groove that runs along either side of the spine. Do five seconds of deep friction massage with your thumbs in this groove, move your hands half an inch further up the body and repeat. Continue doing this until it is no longer possible to reach any further up your back. Then pick up and kneed the large muscles on each side of the spine, beginning on the buttocks and working upwards.

The stomach and lower back mirror tensions elsewhere in the body. The initial spurt of anxiety in a stressful situation is, typically, experienced in the pit of the stomach. It alerts us that we are under strain and usually causes a rapid spread of anxiety symptoms to the rest of the body. The advantage of this massage technique is that it improves the internal functioning of the stomach, which may be disturbed by tension, as well as relaxing the external muscles.

Foot massage

Perhaps the idea of easing away bodily tensions by massaging the feet strikes you as rather strange. In fact this is an especially relaxing technique which affects the whole body, because the feet are focal points for acupressure lines and so transmit stress releasing signals throughout the system.

Foot reflexologists use all kinds of instruments for massaging the feet. For example, to relieve sciatic pains, they use the rubber eraser tip of a pencil to locate a deep point off the centre of the heel pad towards the outside of the foot. And for menstrual cramps the area below the ankle bones is massaged for 30 seconds.

A famous health spa in the USA recommends filling a low heeled pair of lace up shoes with dried peas or beans (e.g. soya) and walking around as long as you can bear, to give yourself your own reflexology foot massage. If you have a particularly tender area, you can check the corresponding organ on a reflexology chart. Rolling your feet back and forward on a coco-cola bottle has the right shape to give your feet a relaxing massage. Also massaging the foot with a small rubber ball works well. Do this all over the foot: inside, outside, on the ball of the foot, the arch, and underneath the toes. Try any of these methods to see which works best for you. The series of massage movements which follow are particularly relaxing after a stressful day.

Foot soothe

Sitting down, rest your left foot on your right knee and apply deep friction massage to the arch for 15 seconds using the heel of the right hand.

Place your thumbs on the arch of the foot, so they are just touching, and stroke in small circles applying moderate pressure. When you reach the centre, pause here and massage upwards towards the ball of the foot. Press and hold for 30 seconds. It will renew your energy. Move the thumbs slowly towards the toes as you do so. The next stage is to apply more deep friction massage, this time using the left thumb only, along the side of the inner border of the foot. Progress from the heel to the base of the big toe.

Now apply deep friction to the ball of the foot, using both thumbs, working upwards to the base of the toe. Continue along the base of the toes. Tension builds up in this area due to both emotional and physical stress. For example if you wear high heels there is likely to be considerable strain in the area around the 3rd and 4th toes.

Turn your foot to work on the upper area. Placing your right thumb on the junction between the first and second toes, start with a gentle deep friction massage lasting about five seconds. Move your thumb a little way along the groove which forms between these toes – it is the space between the tendons – and repeat the massage. Do this until you come to a point where the groove disappears into the foot. Repeat the same massage in the grooves between all the other toes.

Massage each of the toes in turn, as follows. Grasp one toe between your thumb and index finger, then make a gentle, circular, stroking movement almost as if you were attempting to unscrew it! Do not use so much force that you actually twist the toes, rather allow your thumb and finger to slip across the surface of the skin.

Now give each toe a gentle pull. You must not wrench it as this would cause pain, but tenderly and lightly ease it forward.

The last thing I want you to do is place all four fingertips against the ball of the foot, curling them under the centre with your thumbs pointing forwards.

Gently bend the edges of the foot inwards by applying upwards pressure with the fingers and downward force with the thumb pads. There is quite enough elasticity in the foot to allow this movement to occur easily and without the slightest trace of discomfort provided you apply the pressure slowly and smoothly. Now reverse the movement lifting the sides of the foot upwards. Bend and lift the sides of the foot in this way for around ten seconds. When you have finished repeat the whole sequence with your right foot.

At the end of this session of self-massage you should feel deeply relaxed. Carry these sensations into your next activity by getting up slowly and moving in the most relaxed way possible as you set about the tasks ahead.

Enhancing your sensual pleasure

Sexual activity sometimes causes people anxiety and produces stresses which can greatly detract, if not from performance then from the pleasures involved.

The ancient Egyptians found that a few drops of essential oils added to the water in which they bathed just before making love, greatly increased the pleasure and sensuality of both their own and their partner's responses. The same oils were also added to the massage balm, which I have already described. Today, ancient lore has been given a scientific basis by the work of Dr Knutt Larrson of Goteborg University, Sweden, who has found a link between odours and the nerves which control the sexual organs. By stimulating the olfactory system, they also serve to arouse our sensuality.

Prepare a sensual balm by adding a few drops of just *one* of these oils, Jasmine, Carnation or Ylang-Ylang to your basic massage oil. You will find that this heightens both your own sexual enjoyment and your partner's pleasure.

Now for an exercise which will help to tone up the muscles directly involved in love-making.

Acupressure to improve your sexuality

Lie on your back on the floor. Bend your right leg, keeping the foot on the floor, and place the left ankle just above the right knee. Press along the surface of the left thigh which is facing upwards. This movement should be done as near the groin as possible. Continue this for about five minutes and then massage the other thigh in exactly the same manner. Try to time this technique with your breathing by pressing in when you exhale and releasing the pressure when you inhale.

Finish off by pressing gently with the heels of the hands about two inches either side of the navel. Then move your hands down about two inches below the navel and press gently. Pressure on each point should be continued for three minutes, using the breathing and massage timing described above. Finish with effluerage in a clock-wise direction.

You will also find the pelvic lift on page 78 and the stomach soothe on page 118 helpful.

Toning the vaginal muscles

You can do this by sitting cross-legged, or kneeling down and sitting back on your heels. Inhale and, as you breathe out, contract the muscles of the anus, trying to draw them inwards and upwards. Hold this tension, then relax and breathe in again. The contraction of these muscles is only carried out as you exhale. With a little practice you will find that you can contract the muscles of the vagina as you do those of the anus. The back of the vagina is under the control of the same group of the muscles as the front of the anus. You can test your progress by attempting to control the flow of urine by contracting the vaginal muscles. This takes a little time to perfect but you will be able to achieve very good control over the vaginal muscles if you persevere and so greatly enhance the mutual pleasures of love-making.

Toning the erectile muscles

The same exercise can be used to tone up the muscles under the scrotum which are involved in producing an erection.

How to us these techniques

To some extent, the way in which you put those Body Sense

techniques to work for you will be determined by your personal needs. You may, for instance, find that a certain sequence of movements gives the best relief from a particular type of stress and prefer this to the others. Since the nature of stress changes, as do the

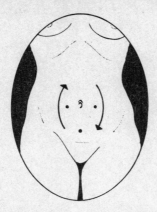

Fig. 87

causes of our stress responses, it may be that a technique which is especially effective at one period of your life becomes less soothing when situations alter and you will then need to adopt a different approach. As a general guide, however, I suggest that you put the techniques to work in the following ways:

Use Thought Stopping, Mind Travel and the Swing-Release to cope with everyday stress problems as they arise. They offer a rapid, convenient and effective method for bringing negative thoughts and needless bodily tensions under control. The Shao Lin technique should be looked on as a natural 'pep-up', to be used any time you feel a bit down or stale. It will raise your spirits and leave you more alert and energetic.

Yeun Chun, the most intricate exercise I have described so far, may deter you at first because of the seeming complexity involved. But I do hope you will give it a try since the feeling of relaxation which results must be experienced to be believed. You can use it to alleviate mental and physical tension during periods of special stress or, if you live most of your life under pressure, as a regular part of your Body Sense health care programme.

The massage techniques should be used in much the same way, and there is no need to wait until the end of the day in order to put them to work. As you become more sensitive to sixth sense messages tension signals will start to receive the attention they deserve and you will want to work to reduce them as quickly as possible, before they start to produce the distressing symptoms of headaches, muscle stiffness and emotional exhaustion. The six quick and convenient soothers described above are the ideal way to cure problems before they arise.

PART FIVE

The Body Sense way to looking good

How you feel about your looks inevitably exerts a powerful influence over the way you look after yourself. Somebody who views themselves very negatively usually lacks interest in taking consistent care of their health. Bad feelings about the body almost always distract attention from bad feelings *within* the body. Look good and you will want to feel good. Feel in excellent health and you are well on your way to looking good as well.

Nobody can hope to be at their best when plagued by physical discomfort and mental distress. By relieving aches and pains, preventing such problems from arising in the first place and learning how to handle stress effectively, you will go a long way towards achieving complete fitness. In this next section of the book I am going to show you some special techniques for staying in peak condition and enjoying what I call whole body health – that radiant sensation of well-being which comes from being mentally and physically on top of the world. All these techniques will, therefore, help you to feel confident about your appearance. The correct posture, graceful ease of movement, clear complexion and a zest for living enormously enhance a person's looks. But, in addition to these indirect rewards for using Body Sense Therapy, I want to tell you how it is possible to restore and rejuvenate your appearance directly. The methods I am going to describe will enable you to put right any harm caused by a previously unhealthy approach to life and prevent such difficulties from undermining your appearance in the future.

This is just as important to men as to women. Thankfully we have moved away from the belief that males who took a sensible interest in their appearance were somehow unmanly. There is absolutely no reason why a desire to look your best should be confined to females, any more than health should be seen as something which only concerns women. It is in everybody's interest for men to remain young and attractive looking no matter what their age. Many of my clients are actors, sportsmen and other personalities who, being so often in the public eye, are naturally concerned with appearances. But they also include a large number of professional people, who realise that by feeling good about themselves they increase the enthusiasm which they bring to their careers, and retain the confidence of their colleagues by looking as good as they feel.

Whole body health means safeguarding the image you present to the outside world no less than protecting your body from the wear and tear of everyday life.

The hidden language of your face

I am going to spend quite a lot of time talking about the face and describing ways in which you can keep your features looking youthfully attractive. Why is it so important to pay special attention to the face? Quite simply because it is the window revealing the way we feel.

When you visit somebody who is ill you tend to say: 'He looked terrible . . .' or 'He looked a good deal better today.' This is because we judge health on the basis of various clues supplied by the way the skin and muscles of the face are working. A poor complexion, which robs the skin of its bloom and gives it a grey, drab appearance is almost always associated with ill-health. When we speak of somebody being 'in the pink' we are actually describing the kind of complexion associated with good health. Similarly a lined, wrinkled face with muscles which sag, or a gaunt, haggard expression are going to tell us of disease and distress.

You will hardly be surprised, therefore, to learn that your face also mirrors emotions very precisely, especially when they are intense. What you may find rather more surprising is the fact that facial muscles also respond to *thoughts* about emotions. Just thinking about being angry or happy, for example, causes the muscles to tense into an appropriate expression – even though we remain quite unaware of these subtle changes.

This powerful but unexpected influence has been demonstrated with dramatic clarity by Harvard psychologist Dr Gary Schwartz in a series of experiments which used very sensitive recording equipment to measure tiny electrical impulses in these muscles. After wiring up a group of volunteers, Dr Schwartz asked his subjects to think about some emotion, to image themselves feeling anxious or aggressive, sad or solemn, carefree or careworn. Although observers were usually unable to detect any changes of expression, and the people concerned were confident that their faces had remained a bland mask throughout, the recording electrodes could not be fooled. They picked up a specific sequence of electrical impulses for each type of emotion. Impulses which, had they been more powerful, would have produced changes of expression consistent with each mental response. Moreover, when the subjects were simply told to think about 'a typical day' their facial muscles hummed like telephone lines with a multitude of messages.

Dr Schwarz's findings indicate that our features are seldom at rest. A busy mind produces millions of hurrying impulses to the muscle groups of the face during the course of a perfectly normal day. This continual, but usually unnoticed, electrical activity has important implications for the way we look, especially when our minds are dominated by a particular emotion.

If you are constantly anxious or depressed, for instance, much of the impulse traffic will set the muscles into expressions appropriate for this mental state. Although our overall expression may not reveal inner despondency, the delicate facial musculature will respond to gloomy thoughts. After a while, constant contractions will produce a 'muscle memory'. That is the pattern of our thoughts will have been noticeably etched into the features. So when we speak of somebody always looking anxious or seeming perpetually gloomy we are actually describing a muscle memory pattern created by months, or perhaps years, of inner uncertainty and depression. These emotions have, as it were, been preserved in a mould of muscle and skin. The wrinkles, lines, and tension marks have created a mask that accurately reflects a particular attitude to life. This need not be a mirror of unhappiness of course. It could equally be a joyful expression or one full of calm assurance.

Because the face has so many hardworking muscles, many of them small and delicate, it runs a special risk of aging prematurely. The way to prevent facial muscles from losing their tone or to limit their harmful effects once the process has begun, is to develop a special sixth sense responsiveness in this area so that you become aware of the way these muscles are working and avoid fixing them into a particular pattern. In addition, you need a knowledge of methods which can be used to ease away tensions and improve the efficiency of the muscles and the circulation. After studying and using a large number of techniques I have found that the ones described below are most effective for this purpose.

Face your face with confidence

The human face has the capacity to respond to the most fleeting changes of mood and thought, but the extent of this responsiveness varies greatly from one person to the next. Some individuals are able to develop a 'poker face' approach to life which successfully masks even quite vigorous signals to the muscles. The majority of faces, however respond fairly uninhibitedly to each passing emotion and, as a result, are more prone to early aging and premature wrinkles.

Just as a body needs regular exercise to remain healthy, so must the face be given frequent attention to keep it looking good. No amount of face creams and make-up can improve inefficient muscle function. Facial exercise and self-massage, however, will both tone up the muscles and improve the flow of blood to the skin, nourishing cells and clearing away the naturally produced poisons which so harm your complexion.

I will start by describing a series of easily performed facial exercises which serve this purpose admirably. They should be carried out once each day, take no more than five minutes to complete and are suitable both for men and women.

Throat and chin

(1) I want you to start by imagining there is an apple suspended on a thread just above your nose. Tilt back your head and bite vigorously at it working your jaws hard as if nibbling pieces off. This is a great warming up exercise and will send the blood rushing to your chin and neck muscles.

After about 12 bites stop with your mouth wide open and turn up the corners of the mouth in an exaggerated smile. Hold this position and count slowly to six. As you slowly close the mouth make sure you maintain the smiling position. Relax and repeat twice more.

(2) Lie down on the bed, with your shoulders supported, and your

head hanging over the edge. Relax completely. Very slowly bring your head so that the chin touches your chest. Then, just as slowly, return to the starting position. At first I suggest you only repeat this movement three times. With practice, however, you will find it quite simple to build up to twelve repetitions.

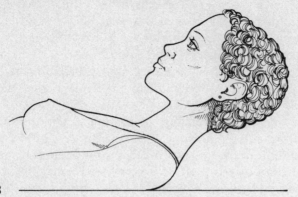

Fig. 88

(3) For the final exercise here, cup your chin in your hands with the fingers resting on the sides of the cheeks, and the heels of the hands under the chin, turn up the corners of your mouth. Now attempt to open your mouth while resisting the movement. Hold the tension for a slow count of seven and relax. Repeat this three times.

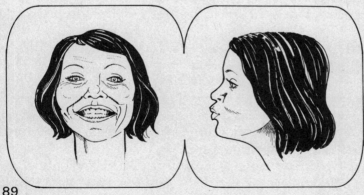

Fig. 89

Cheeks and lips

(1) You should start with your lips together. Give an exaggerated grin, turning the corners of the mouth up as high as you can. Take a

slow count of seven to reach the highest point of this movement. Then push the muscles completely forward, without losing the upward pull. Hold for a slow count of seven. Slowly relax and repeat three times.

(2) Again, with your lips together, swing them across the face and up to the other side to tense the cheek muscles. Hold for a slow count of seven. Do this on both sides of the face. Relax.

(3) Now cupping your hands under the cheekbones push upwards while you contract the muscles for a slow count of seven. This was the favourite exercise of a famous oriental beauty who always completed it by *very light* rapid pinching movements over the entire face and neck.

Form an 'O' with your lips, flattening them, pulling and contracting hard the circular band of muscle that holds them in shape. Maintain the tension, as before, to a slow count of seven. This is an especially important exercise if you smoke, since the action of holding a cigarette between your lips creates wrinkles around them.

Finally puff out your cheeks as hard as you can, count slowly to seven and relax. As you do this flatten your lips otherwise you will create small wrinkles with your upper lip.

Eyes

Eye exercises will help preserve the youthful appearance of the very delicate skin in this part of the face, skin which can easily lose its tone and start to sag in a most unattractive manner by early middle-age.

Start by opening your eyes as wide as possible. Press your fingertips against your forehead to prevent wrinkling while doing this exercise. Hold for the usual slow count of seven.

Now place your palms over your eyes, with the thumbs resting in the small hollows at each temple. Squeeze the eyes closed, at the same time resisting this movement with your thumbs. As before hold the tension for a slow count to seven.

Finally, with your eyes wide open, place three fingers *gently* on the cheek bone and against this *slight* resistance try to raise your lower lid towards the upper lid. Count slowly to seven as you strive towards the maximum eyelid raise. At seven relax slowly and repeat the exercise three times on each side of the face.

Forehead

Wrinkles here are sometimes thought of as giving men an 'intellectual' appearance. They are simply indications that the muscles have been forced into a mould by holding one expression for too long. Tone up your forehead muscles to help banish wrinkles and prevent more from developing, like this.

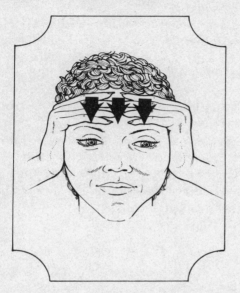

Fig. 90

Start by lifting your forehead, stroking it lightly with the flat of your hand. At the top of the lift place the hand flat against the skull and hold the forehead raise by firm pressure against the bone. Now try to pull the forehead downwards by tensing the muscles against the pull of this pressure. Hold for a slow count of seven as usual.

Next, place the heel of your hand on the forehead between the eyes where scowl lines tend to develop and imagine that those muscles are trying to force your hand away. Hold for the usual slow count of seven.

From exercises to help prevent loss of muscle tone, we move to a series of massages which will bring fresh blood supplies to the surface areas of the face so keeping the complexion looking good. After carrying out this self-massage your face should feel warm and refreshed. It will be more relaxed and the harmful effects of muscle contraction which I described in my introduction to this section will be guarded against. To prevent friction between your hands and face you should start by spreading a thin layer of your favourite cream or oil onto your face.

Face massage

Chin, throat and upper cheek

The first massage takes in the throat and upper chest because most people overlook these two areas in their routine beauty care. A massage given by a professional, however, will always include them because, although not part of the face itself, they detract from facial beauty if allowed to become unattractive. They form a kind of pedestal for the face and anybody looking at you cannot help but be aware of them.

Massage these areas as follows: Make sure your movements are firm but light enough not to stretch the skin. You can avoid stretching the skin by tensing the muscles you are massaging and thus exercising the face at the same time. Cup both hands and place them on the jawbone at the chin.

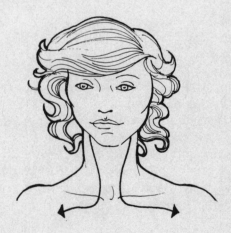

Fig. 91

Keeping your hands in this cupped position stroke down the side of the neck, following the arrows in Figure 91, below the neck and along the décolleté. Do this eight times applying gentle pressure.

The next stage is to place the sides of your index fingers along the groove of your chin with your thumbs just below the jawbone, as shown in Figure 92. Maintaining this position gently squeeze the thumbs and fingers together. Move half an inch along the chin and squeeze again. Continue like this until you reach the end of the jawbone. Repeat eight times.

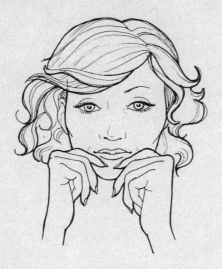

Fig. 92

Now place the backs of the fingers of both hands under the chin and make a rapid 'fluttering' movement with your fingers, bringing them up to strike the skin with the backs of as many fingers as you can. Do this with both hands at once for about ten seconds.

In the next massage sequence you use your knuckles to stimulate the skin and muscles. Make a fist, and move the flat surface of the knuckles of each finger in turn against the skin, starting with the little finger. Use both hands at the same time and move all over the front of the neck and down on the décolleté for about 20 seconds.

Now do 'knuckling', in exactly the same way as before, from the middle of the underside of the chin moving out along the neck to the ears. Move slowly. It should take about 20 seconds to complete this massage. When doing knuckling tense the muscles so as not to stretch the skin. Repeat twice more. Oriental beauties knew thousands of years ago to press on a point near the thyroid to retain that beauty. Hold 3 seconds. Repeat four times on each side of the neck, as in Figure 93.

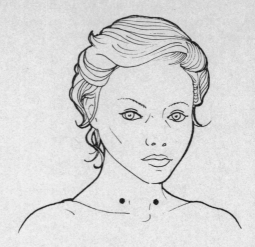

Fig. 93

Cheeks and lips

Start by placing the fingers of each hand at the corners of the mouth. Stroke outwards and upwards towards the ears. Repeat this ten times.

Next place the fingertips of each hand on the cheeks and, starting with the little fingers, tap the cheeks with one finger at a time. Do this for about 30 seconds moving all over the face, but avoid any areas where there are signs of broken capillaries – that is little red veins in the skin.

For the next massage you are going to use the deep friction technique which you may already have used. If you have not yet done so, or if you are unsure of the method, then turn to page 65 for a reminder of the proper way to carry out this procedure.

Using the forefingers of each hand apply deep friction along the lines shown in the next illustration. Move slowly along the folds – known as the *nasolabial folds* – and continue right up to the sides of the nose. Massage with both hands at once, moving the fingers together. Don't forget to tense the muscles to avoid stretching the skin.

Now do a deep friction massage along the lip line, as shown by the arrow in the next illustration. This should normally take about 15 seconds, but if you smoke regularly you would be advised to

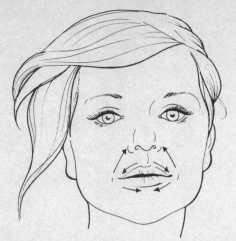

Fig. 94

stimulate this area for a longer period, say 30 seconds in order to help eliminate the strains which holding a cigarette places on the lip muscles.

For the final cheeks and lips massage place the forefingers of both hands above the lips and the middle fingers just beneath the lips. Sweep the hands suddenly outwards at the same time squeezing the lips together. Repeat this ten times.

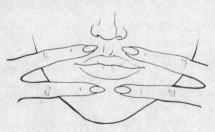

Fig. 95

Forehead

Start by placing the fingertips of both hands on the forehead with the tips of the little fingers resting on the eyebrows. Stroke upwards and outwards pressing with moderate firmness. Carry out a little deep friction with the fingertips between the eyebrows to control scowl lines. Repeat ten times.

Next I want you to place the forefinger and middle finger of the left hand on the centre of the forehead, keeping the fingers slightly spread. Place the forefinger of the right hand between these two fingers so that the tip of the right finger is lined up with the tips of the left fingers, as shown in Figure 96. Now make a series of rapid movements, pushing the hands towards one another and then away again. Do this for 20 seconds all over the forehead. Finish by briskly tapping all over the forehead as you did the cheeks.

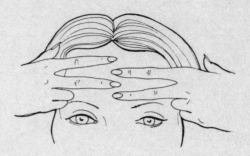

Fig. 96

Eyes

Finally you should gently press and slowly rotate the middle fingers of each hand in the hollows near the corners of the eyes. Do this for about five seconds. Next circle the middle fingers slowly along the under edge of the eye-sockets. Move up and around until you reach the inner edge of the eyebrows. At this point you will find

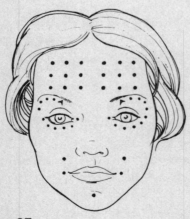

Fig. 97a

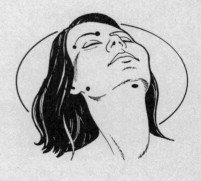

Fig. 97b

two small hollows (marked with arrows in Figure 97a). Press here for three seconds. Then continue to circle around the top of the eyesocket. Make at least ten circles around the perimeter of the socket. Now tense the muscles around the eye and press with the fingertips of four fingers for a count of seven seconds above and below the eyes.

This Shiatzu facial massage will improve the condition of your skin and muscle tone of your face. Spread your fingers out and press on the points on the forehead shown in the Figure 97a. Use the first three fingers of both hands, and press on each set of points for ten seconds. Repeat twice more. This procedure helps to prevent wrinkles in the forehead.

Now press two-three minutes on the points in Figure 97b. The drawing shows the right half of the face, but the points are located in the same spots on the other side of the face, so you should also press there.

That is, press for two minutes at the points on the outer corners of the eyes. Then press for two minutes at the outer and inner ends of the eyebrows. You will feel a tiny notch on these points. Finally, press for two minutes with the thumb on the points under the chin and in the recess of the chin.

Dry, scaly skin is a common problem which can give an appearance of poor health even if you actually feel quite fit. As new skin cells are formed they gradually travel upwards to the surface where they flatten out into flaky scales. These are automatically shed to make way for new, young looking cells essential for a good complexion. As we get older this process slows down and nature may need a little help in order to send the worn out, unattractive, cells on their way. This need has long been recognised by many cultures and a number of patent remedies exist. The Indians use ground seeds and nuts mixed into a paste, for example; Polynesians the loofah plant, Arabs use sand and the Japanese sea sponges. One of the best methods I know is finely ground corn meal which can be used in the bath or the shower. Massage it vigorously into the skin to slough off unwanted cells. If your skin is especially dry, use a mixture of olive oil and sea salt instead.

Now lets consider complexion in rather more detail, and in particular a condition known as cellulite or orange-peel skin from the fact that, if you push up a small portion of the skin it has the lumpy appearance of orange skin.

How to banish cellulite

The starting point must be diet. Keep it low in fat and sugar, except for the naturally occurring sugars. Eat plenty of fruit and vegetables raw and in salads, especially those which stimulate the production of urine, since cellulite is largely due to fluid retention. You *should* eat: cucumbers, which are the greatest natural diuretic. Also good are green beans, leeks, onions, celery, bean sprouts, parsley and fennel. Avoid eating too much meat, but take plenty of raw salads and vegetables with a little grilled or baked chicken or fish. Cut out salt entirely and use only herbs to flavour your meals.

Drink approximately two pints of bottled mineral water a day, some immediately on rising and the rest between meals.

As an extra way to banish cellulite, Maurice Messegue, the famous French herbalist, recommends ground ivy leaves either crushed and rubbed into the skin, or applied as a poultice for several hours. Other herbalists recommend violet leaves.

Cellulite self-massage

Start with slow effleurage on the area in which the cellulite occurs, gradually increasing the speed. Follow this with petrissage on the area, moving upward in an S-shaped pattern. Unlike the petrissage I recommend for sore muscles, with cellulite you should do it in a superficial manner, making sure you do not massage too deeply or heavily.

Twist into the cellulite with your fingertips or knuckles, giving a short sharp pull in an upward direction until the whole area is covered. Now carry out 'plucking' on the affected part with the middle finger and thumb. Plucking means taking hold of a piece of the flesh between the thumb and middle finger and giving it a light quick twist and releasing. The movement should be very light and rapid with the accent upwards.

Massage can be enhanced if you use a lubricant consisting of one cup of soya oil; 8 drops of essential oil of sage; 2 drops of essential oil of juniper. These oils counteract fluid retention. When taking a bath or shower use a friction glove or loofah to stimulate the skin. If these procedures are followed you should find that cellulite will be measureably improved.

Bear in mind the comments I made in the last part of the book when talking about stress. Emotional upheavals are very, very often reflected in the complexion. You must work at reducing tension and stress while enhancing your appearance.

Excess weight

If you are overweight you might be interested in experimenting with the two techniques below which are said to suppress appetite. Both rely on the discovery of particular pressure points. The first lies at a point located halfway between the nose and upper lip. Hold your upper lip between your thumb and index finger and massage for a minute.

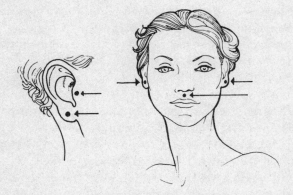

Fig. 98

The other two pressure points are in the ear. Stimulate these points with the end of a matchstick or tooth pick when tempted to overeat.

When you have achieved your desired weight you should work hard at toning your muscles with the isometric exercises in Part 6. Meanwhile, here is a herbal lotion for toning up the flabby skin that almost inevitably results from loss of weight. Bring to the boil a litre of mineral water. Let it cool a little before adding 10 grammes each of lavender flowers, blackberry leaves, nettle and celandine. Let the mixture steep overnight, strain and use while still freshly made. Spray the mixture on the skin with a plant sprayer if possible. Rub the mixture briskly into the skin.

To complete this section of the Body Sense approach to looking your best, I am going to describe a technique for developing firmer, more shapely breasts by building the pectoral muscles. This usually gives a boost to a woman's confidence about her looks as well as bringing about actual physical improvement.

Male readers who are unhappy with their chest development can also use this technique for improving the size, shape and firmness of these important muscles. Even men who do not have the slightest desire to resemble a 'Mr Universe', usually wish they looked a little more imposing when stripped to the waist or wearing swimming trunks. By this technique they can achieve their ambition without any need for weights or chest expanders.

The method I shall describe was discovered some two thousand years ago by the Chinese. A subtle combination of muscle tension and special breathing it provides one of the fastest and most effective aids to building a more attractive body that I have ever discovered.

The Chinese named it the Tong Long, or praying mantis because the position of the hands resembles the prayerful attitude adopted by that insect as it waits for its prey.

How to do the tong long

Stand with arms stretched out straight and held at a slight angle to the body. Fingers are extended, palms face downwards.

Hunch your shoulders forward slightly and begin to move the elbows very slowly inwards towards an imaginary spot about one inch above the navel. As you do this tense the chest muscles and those in your arms as tightly as possible. When you have achieved the correct amount of tension you will begin to feel the arm muscles vibrating slightly while those around the breasts will grow rigid and tight. This rigidity is essential to the success of the exercise. Without it no toning of muscles or tissue development can take place.

When you are sure your chest muscles are tight continue to move your elbows, as slowly as possible, towards the imaginary spot above the navel. While doing this, slowly close your hands into fists and turn your palms until they are facing upwards. This aids the contraction of the other muscles which we are building by this exercise.

The final position is shown in Figure 94. By the end of the exercise your forearms will be touching and your elbows resting against the

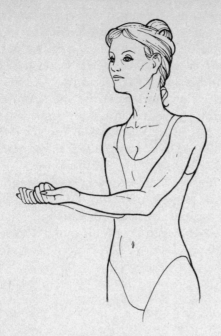

Fig. 99

spot on your stomach just above the navel. Hold this at full tension for a couple of seconds.

Now *snap* your arms outward and upward returning to the starting position ready to begin another repetition of the movements.

The *snap* movement is important and should be performed very rapidly because the *sudden release* of all the tension contributes almost as much to building firm muscle tissue as the tension itself.

When carrying out this exercise correct breathing is extremely important. From the starting position half fill your lungs. As you inhale make sure the chest does not expand at all. Instead move your stomach outwards while breathing in. Imagine that it contains a large balloon which is drawing the air down through your nose and lungs.

When the balloon is full move to the second part of the exercise breathing out slowly through the mouth. As you thrust your arms outward and turn and open your hands suddenly, exhale through your mouth the air that remains in your imaginary abdominal balloon. Breathe in again and you are ready to do another repetition. The Chinese who developed this ancient exercise found that breathing like this *doubles* muscle expansion.

Carry out this exercise five times a week. After each five day session allow two days free of exercise so that the tissues have time to build up. This is included in your programme. At first carry out around 20 repetitions a day then, as you become more practised, increase to 40 each day. After around a fortnight there will be a noticeable increase in breast size and firmness. Eight weeks continuous exercise should add several inches to your measurements.

The Oriental races massage the bosom gently to keep it firm and shapely. Carry out petrissage on the pectoral muscles just close to the armpit. Massage the bosom with circular outward effleurage. Use a few drops of a light citrus scented oil such as lemon grass added to your base oil.

PART SIX

The Body Sense way to lasting health

If your muscles and connective tissues are in peak condition then your whole body will look good and you will feel alert and energetic. The secret of long lasting fitness, therefore, depends on sustaining the quality of these vital but seldom considered parts of the body.

So far, I have told you how your inner powers of self-healing can be used to prevent or relieve aches and pains, to counter the effects of stress and to enhance your appearance, so giving you self-confidence when facing the world. In this part of the book, I am going to tell you how these same, potent forces for health can be used to strengthen your body's defences against infection, to increase stamina and to prolong youthful vigour. All the procedures you will learn are easy to use and make few demands on the busiest schedule, indeed one of them can be fitted into any odd moment during the day while another takes little more than a minute to complete. They are drawn from a variety of ancient and modern sources, but united by their ability to draw on your natural reserves of health giving power.

As with a number of the Body Sense techniques we have looked at already, these take longer to explain and to read than they do to put into action. I suggest you read through each of them and use the illustrations to gain a general understanding of the techniques involved. As you begin to use them, move slowly through the sequence of movements until your knowledge and confidence are sufficient to allow a rapid progression through the different stages. I am going to start by explaining how to enhance a part of the circulatory system which is, I suspect, almost unknown outside the medical profession. Yet your health is vitally dependent on its effective function. The fluid being moved around the body is called lymph and the network of tubes through which it is transported is termed the lymphatic system.

Draining the lymphatic system

Lymph is an odourless, watery, slightly yellowish fluid whose job it is to transport material between the blood and cells. By means of the lymphatic system these cells are provided with food for energy and able to get rid of the waste products which build up as they work. If we get an infection, poison gathers in the lymph glands – located at various points around the body – which become tender and swollen. This swelling and tenderness is one of the first signs your doctor will look for if he suspects you have contracted an infection.

Even from this brief description of its functions, the importance of a healthy lymphatic system should become clear. It is just as vital to the body's physical fitness as uninterrupted food supplies and an efficient sewerage system is to the health of a great city. Only when the drainage is working correctly can the cells flourish. Poor lymphatic circulation leads to starved and weakened tissue being polluted and destroyed by its own waste products. That is why I believe the massage which assists this drainage, a technique developed from research carried out in Denmark, is one of the most vital you will ever learn in Body Sense Therapy.

Why do we need to give the lymph a helping hand? The main reason is that, unlike the blood, lymph has no regularly pumping heart to move it about the body. Instead, its circulation depends on a constant squeezing action by the muscles. If you lead a somewhat sedentary life – and most people do these days – then the muscles may not work hard enough to circulate the lymph adequately. As a result, its progress is sluggish, some cells receive insufficient attention and poisons tend to accumulate in various parts of the body. The Danish physiotherapists who pioneered the treatment have shown that, by carrying out this drainage massage as part of a regular programme of health care, the lymph can be kept flowing freely and cell health, on which our own health ultimately depends, maintained at peak levels. Once lymphatic congestion has been eliminated the cells receive all the nutrients needed for natural functioning and are cleansed of their harmful by-products. After carrying out the massage for only a few weeks you will probably be astonished at how much more alert and energetic you feel. As well as stimulating the lymph flow, this technique also works to get rid of excess bodily fluid, an important cause of people looking and feeling overweight.

How to perform the massage

All the movements have to be made *in the direction of the lymph glands* so that the fluid is drained towards them. It is important, for this reason, to follow my instructions exactly and only stroke or massage your body in the way I describe.

You should undress down to your underclothes and sit on your bed with your back well supported. Make sure the room is warm enough for comfort. You may find it helpful to keep a blanket beside you to cover those parts of the body not being massaged.

Make your muscles more receptive to the treatment by closing your eyes and relaxing as deeply as possible for a few minutes. When you are ready to begin start at the lowest extremity by moving the lymph upwards from your feet.

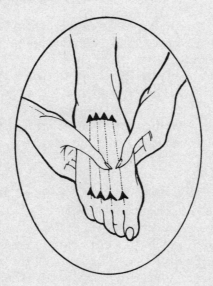

Fig. 100

Feet massage

Bend your right knee up and place the fingers of both hands under the arch of the right foot. Starting between the first and second toes, use your thumbs to stroke back along the grooves between the tendons on the upper side of the foot. Do four strokes with each thumb using a medium pressure. Now repeat exactly the same movements, this time working on the tendons running back from the third and fourth toes.

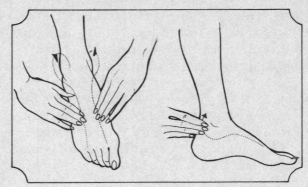

Fig. 101

Place your hands in the V-position illustrated in Figure 101. Stroke backwards firmly with both hands so that the fingers pass first under and behind the ankle bone on both sides (as indicated by the arrows). Do eight strokes on each foot in turn. Massage around the ankle bones both inside and outside the foot using deep friction.

When the massage to the right foot is complete switch to the left foot and carry out exactly the same movements as before.

Lower legs massage

Now move up the body to tackle the lymph system in the lower legs. Place the heels of the hands on the right leg, just over the ankle with one hand on each side as shown in the next illustration. Press firmly with the heels of both hands simultaneously so that they stroke around the back of the leg in a movement which is upwards and slightly diagonal, as shown by the arrows. The heels of the hands should meet at the back of the leg on the completion of each stroke. Carry out one stroke, move the hands about one inch up the leg and repeat. Continue in this way overlapping the strokes until you reach the knee.

Next, grasp the right ankle with the right hand, thumb on the

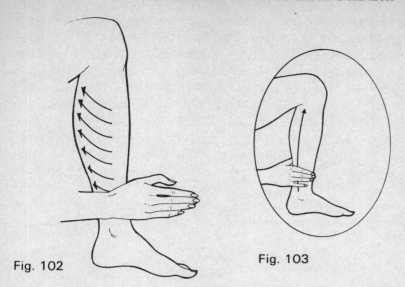

Fig. 102   Fig. 103

inside and fingers on the outside, as shown in Figure 103. Stroke up
the calf applying a firm pressure to the back of the leg.

Grasp the right ankle as before, and, using your *left* hand, stroke
firmly upwards. Continue this movement alternating hands. Carry
on doing this until you have completed *eight* repetitions on the right
leg. Then repeat the whole procedure on the left leg. By doing this
massage you will have eased the lymph up from the toes towards the
thighs which is the next area of the body to receive attention.

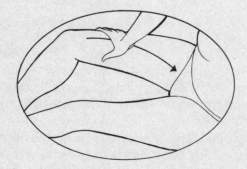

Fig. 104

Thighs massage

This can be carried out most easily if you remain seated on the bed
but have the leg concerned resting on a bedside stool. Bend the right

knee and grasp your thigh with the right hand so that the thumb is on the inside and the fingers against the outside as shown in Figure 104. Press firmly with thumb, fingers and the heel of the hand and stroke upwards and inwards towards the groin. This is shown by the arrow in Figure 104. Note also that it is the *heel of the hand* which does most of the work here and should be held down with a firm pressure.

Now rest the heel of the *left hand* on the top of the right thigh, close to the knee. The fingers are on the inside of the thigh, the thumb rests against the outside and the heel of the hand applies pressure to the top of the muscle. Press firmly and stroke towards the groin as before.

Using alternate hands as you did when massaging the lower leg, repeat eight times and do the same type of movements on the left thigh.

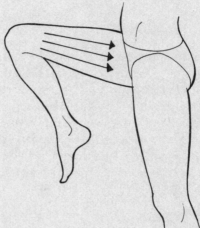

Fig. 105

To massage the inner thigh you use a very similar sequence of alternate right and left hand movements. Begin, as before, by working on the right leg. Grasp the inner part of the thigh with your right hand, thumb above and fingers below. Stroke towards the groin. After one complete stroke switch to the left hand, this time the thumb will be pointing downwards while the fingers curve towards the top of the leg. Alternate the hands, making eight complete movements with each. Be gentle when carrying out this massage because the inner thighs are usually very sensitive.

The final area to receive attention is the underside of the thigh. To carry out this massage you will need to bend your leg up to your chest. Start, as before, with your right leg. Place the inner part of the forearm against the underside of the thigh, close to the knee. Clasp the right wrist with the left hand.

Pressing firmly with the forearm, move the right arm along the underside of the thigh working diagonally upwards towards the groin in the direction of the arrow. Roll the forearm towards the body during this movement, again, as indicated by the arrows. Carry out this procedure eight times. Repeat entire procedure on left thigh.

Stomach and groin massage

Sit on the bed with your knees bent. Place both hands on your stomach in a V-shaped position as illustrated in Figure 106.

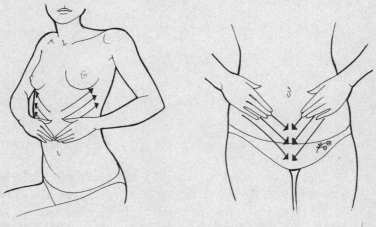

Fig. 106   Fig. 107

The fingers should meet just above the navel while the heels of the hands must rest either side of the abdomen just below the ribcage. Using both hands together stroke upwards and outwards along the lines shown, applying a moderate pressure with the heels of the hands. Stroke towards the armpits, the location of an important lymph gland, and repeat the movements eight times.

Rest the heels of both hands on the hipbones with the fingers pointing towards the groin. Press *gently* with the heels of the hands and stroke downwards to the genitals. Repeat this movement *four times*.

Buttocks massage

Stand up and clench your hands into fists. Place your fists together, so that the knuckles are in contact, at the base of the spine just above the division of the buttocks. Apply a firm pressure stroke with the fists in the direction of the arrows shown in Figure 108. Your fists will each move up a U-shape, curving up around the hips and then down into the groin. Repeat this movement eight times.

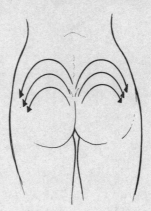

Fig. 108

Hands massage

Sit down again on the bed. To massage the lymph circulation in the hands, proceed in much the same way as I described for the feet. Grasp the right hand with the left, placing the left thumb between the ring and little fingers. Stroke upwards between the tendons which extend away from the ring and little fingers towards the wrist. Repeat this movement four times using moderate pressure. Then change to the tendons which go back from the ring and middle fingers. Stroke upwards four times as before, using moderate pressure. Repeat the same movements between the tendons of the index and middle fingers, and then index finger and thumb. Repeat each of the movements on the left hand using the right thumb.

Arms massage

If you are right handed I advise you to start this procedure by working on the left arm so that you can get the idea of what is needed while using your preferred hand. If you usually work with the left hand then start on the right arm.

Assuming that you are starting work on the left side of the body, proceed as follows. Grasp the left wrist with the right hand so that your fingers and thumb are resting against the outside of the arm.

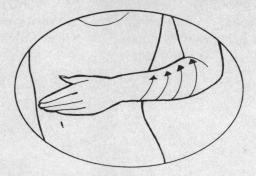

Fig. 109

Applying pressure with the heel of the hands, perform a series of circular movements, stroking the forearm diagonally and inwards as you do so. Follow the arrows in the illustration above. Continue upwards until you reach the crook of the arm. Apply firm pressure throughout, moulding the hand to the forearm. Then stroke firmly up the inside of the forearm from the wrist to the crook of the arm several times. Repeat the movements on other forearm.

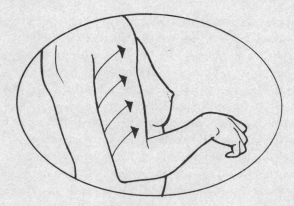

Fig. 110

Start the third arm technique by bringing your right arm across the body, level with your stomach. Then take hold of the upper part of this arm just above the elbow, with the thumb, fingers, and heel of hand. The heel of the hand should be resting against the triceps muscle which lies along the rear of the upper arm. As before, make a circular movement with the hand, while moving slowly diagonally upwards and inwards. Apply firm pressure with the heel of the hand and progress gradually up the arm after each movement until you reach the shoulder. Then stroke firmly up the inside of the upperarm towards the armpit. Do this several times and then repeat the whole procedure on the left upper arm.

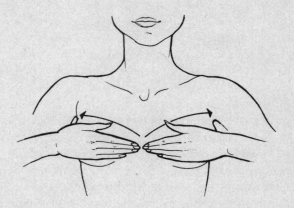

Fig. 111

Chest massage

The final massage improves drainage of lymph in the chest. Sitting up in bed, place both hands on the ribcage very slightly below the level of the armpits. The middle fingers should be touching. Exert a moderate pressure with the heels of both hands simultaneously while moving them towards the armpits in the direction shown by the arrows. Repeat eight times.

This completes the lymphatic drainage technique. Like many other exercises in the book it takes longer to describe than to perform, so do not be put off if the movements appear a little involved on first reading. This massage helps ensure that your cells receive adequate nourishment and function at peak efficiency. By removing their waste products promptly and thoroughly, a smoothly flowing lymphatic system helps you to look and feel healthier. A good time to carry out the technique is after a bath or shower, or just before going to sleep. It will put your body in better condition for a night of restful recuperation.

The no-effort exercise programme

Let me tell you about a client of mine, a company director in his early forties, who suddenly realised he was far from fit. He decided to take up jogging, bought a track suit and running shoes and, full of enthusiasm, set off at the crack of dawn on the first day. His eagerness lasted about a week. Sheer determination kept him going for another ten days, then began to find excuses for missing the daily jogging session. It was difficult to spare the time, he felt too exhausted afterwards to concentrate on his work, it was unpleasant turning out in the rain and so on. A month later he was still *talking* about the need for taking more exercise to stay in trim. But talk was all he was doing. Jogging could have helped him towards health very well indeed had he managed to sustain his interest in regular exercise. But, like the vast majority of people who resolve to improve their fitness, ambition was never transformed into attainment. The truth is that most weight training equipment – stationary bicycles, rowing machines and running shoes and the like – exhaust their owner's motivation long before they themselves get worn out. The value of the keep-fit equipment gathering dust in the backrooms and cupboards of Europe and America must run into millions of pounds!

Let's be realistic. You are probably a very busy person and your time is at a premium. If you are presented with a way of keeping healthy which makes too great an inroad into that already tight routine you may start the programme but I'll take a bet you never finish it. Under the pressures of daily life you miss one exercise session, than another. You promise: 'I'll start again when things get easier.' But of course things never do and you never start again. In the end you give up any real expectation of enjoying total fitness and learn to live with a body that is less than completely efficient and entirely healthy.

I am keenly aware of these difficulties because many of my clients live under constant pressures, with demands that must be satisfied and responsibilities that cannot be avoided. Indeed one of the main reasons why I developed these techniques was to find a way around such problems. So how can the Body Sense way to whole body health help you find the time to stay fit?

The exercises I am going to talk about will build muscle health quickly and effortlessly. They can be fitted into odd moments during the day, and indeed some of them can be carried out in public with no one but yourself being any the wiser. So I am not asking you to find extra time in an already busy schedule. The second important factor is that the exercises are not strenuous.

Often I find that it is the idea of being completely exhausted after a period of vigorous activity, such as squash, swimming or jogging, that puts people off exercising. I am certainly not decrying such activities. They improve your fitness in many important ways, building up the heart, lungs and circulation, improving stamina and helping you to look good as well. But at the start, when you are out of training and relatively unfit, the prospect of tough exercise may prove so daunting that you never begin. As you get back into shape, using my easy, no-effort exercises, you are *more* likely to want to move on to some sport which does make greater demands on your body. But you can approach that point gradually, by paddling around in the shallow end and getting your strength, confidence and interest to a level sufficient to make you want to strike out into deeper waters. If that point is never reached do not worry. The exercise methods I am going to describe are all you really need to feel and look in good shape. Pick whichever of the three techniques suggested is most convenient and agreeable to you. But start using it right away!

Do it to music

Many people find it fun to exercise to music. The beat helps them develop a smooth rhythm that transforms the slog of keeping fit into the fun of the dance floor. Switch on your record player and put on a disco record, or the latest rock music, anything which has a steady beat. The exercises I am about to describe are used for jazz dancing.

Get an upright chair and stand behind it, hands resting on the back. Now move your left foot behind you as far as it will go with the toes on the floor. Put your weight onto the right foot, bend at the knee and bounce your left heel to the floor eight times. Change legs and repeat. This is especially good for overcoming the bunched calf muscles caused by high heels.

Next stand with your legs apart and arms straight up over your head, palms facing outwards. Bend your right knee, stretching your right arm and the right side of your body upwards as much as

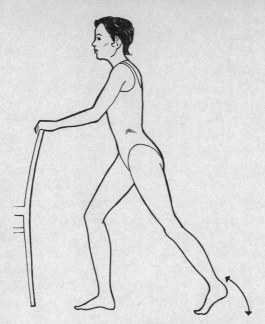

Fig. 112

possible, continue the stretch right through to your fingertips. Next do the same thing on the left side of the body. Keep alternating sides in time to the music. See Figure 113.

Bend at the waist, letting your body drop. Swing your arms through your legs and back out again, as you do this try to get a bounce into your body. On each bounce your arms should swing through your legs and out again. Do this four times. Now go back and repeat the previous two exercises.

Still with your legs apart, toes facing forwards, place your arms straight out to the side, as shown in Figure 115, and lift the ribcage as much as you can. Pretend that your chest is detached from the waist and move it to the right and the left repeatedly for about half a minute.

Now bend your legs and circle the hips. Thrust your right hip to the right; your bottom back; your left hip to the left and finally push your pelvis forward, tucking in the tailbone. Continue for about half a minute. Finally blend these movements together so that you are rotating your hips smoothly in a circle.

The next exercise works on the muscles of the back and shoulders. Stand behind the chair, about four feet away, bend at the waist, and

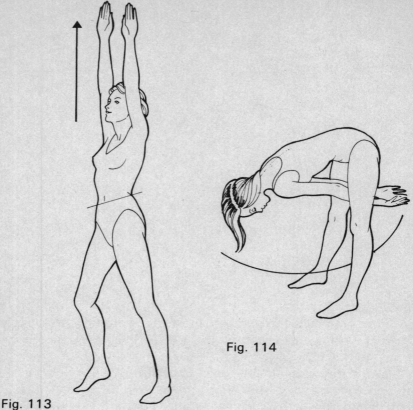

Fig. 114

Fig. 113

place your hands some twelve inches apart on the chair's back. Without bending your knees or arms, flatten your back by pushing it downwards as shown in Figure 117. Now arch your back like a cat, lifting your body upwards as shown in Figure 118. Finally, slowly sink back to the original position. This exercise should be carried out in a smooth, continuous motion. Do this sequence eight times.

The final exercise works on the stomach muscles and pelvis. Stand so that your weight is on the left foot with both knees bent. Push out your backside and arch your back and lift your chin as shown in Figure 119. Now pretend that somebody has hit you in the stomach. Contract the abdominal muscles and tuck in your tailbone and drop your head. Draw your body upwards until both knees are straight.

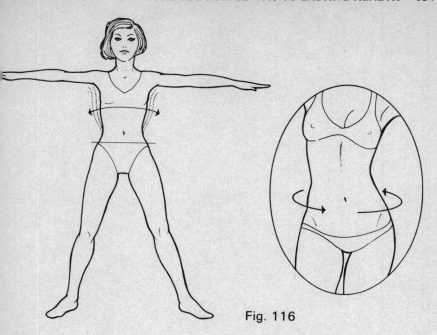

Fig. 116

Fig. 115

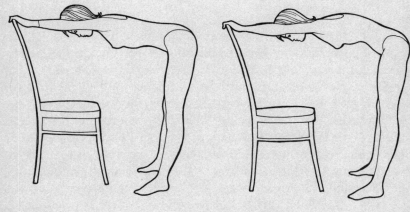

Fig. 117

Fig. 118

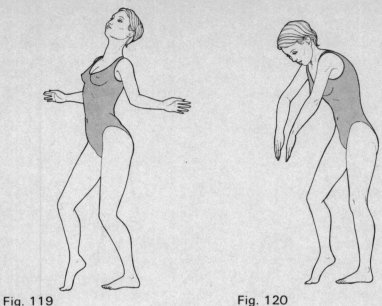

Fig. 119   Fig. 120

Go back to the first movement, that is arching your back and pushing out your bottom, and repeat the whole sequence over and over again for as long as you find comfortable. Incidentally this looks terrific on the disco floor when done as a continuous rippling movement.

Do it in 63 seconds . . .

Here is a series of isometric exercises which will tone and firm up the muscles improving both looks and health. If you have complained in the past that you never have the time to take better care of yourself, the excuses stop here. This sequence of movements gives good muscle tone in just 63 seconds a day! You do not need to take any more time than this because each of the seven-second exercises achieves its maximum effect within the brief period. Research has shown that applying tension to muscles for longer than seven seconds leads to little further improvement in their firmness and tone. You see, by contracting your muscles regularly to their full potential, you will find that this potential increases with each exercise session, resulting in steadily improving muscle strength and tone.

Movement one: For this exercise you will need an ordinary dining room chair. Sit on the floor with your legs stretched out between the legs of the chair and toes pointing upwards. Press outwards against the chair legs as hard as possible. This tones the outer thighs and hips.

Movement two: Place your legs outside the legs of the chair and press inwards. This prevents flabby inner thighs.

Movement three: Now sit on the chair and press your hands firmly together, elbows out to the side. Clasp them and pull them in opposite directions as hard as possible. Hold both the push and the pull for seven seconds.

Movement four: For this movement go to a doorway and place your outstretched arms through the entrance, touching the frame with your wrists. Press outwards as though forcing the door frame apart. It is a wonderful way of preventing flabby upper arms.

Movement five: Sit on the chair with your legs stretched out and place your hands just above the knees. Press down with your hands and up with your legs. This tenses the stomach muscles and you should feel the strain in them.

Movement six: Lie face down on the floor put your legs together and raise your bottom as much as possible without also lifting your back.

Movement seven: Turn face down on the floor and lift your arms and legs off the ground. This is good for toning the muscles of the upper back, bottom and stomach.

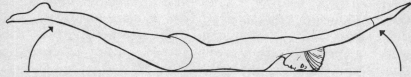

Fig. 121

Carry out each of these movements for just seven seconds, in the order given. Do them each morning and, even if you cannot spare the time for any other exercises, you will quickly discover greater strength and improved muscle tone.

Do it in no time at all . . .

We all have those frantic days when there is simply no time for anything except rushing from one chore to another. At moments like this there seems no hope of giving our bodies the benefit of any muscle-enhancing exercise. But it can be done. For emergencies like this I have developed a simple set of movements which can be done at any odd moments during the day – while waiting for a lift perhaps, standing in a bus queue, or at the sink, during a coffee break, or in the moments before a meeting. It is so discrete that nobody else need know you are exercising and no equipment is needed. Yet it works very effectively to keep you trim and fit. There are just six movements to remember and each needs to be held, as in the previous set of exercises, for seven seconds.

Start by pulling in your stomach muscles as hard as you can. But keep breathing normally. Then tense the muscles of your buttocks as much as possible. Now contract the muscles of the groin and anus as tightly as you can. This is an important lower pelvis exercise which should also improve your sex life.

Curl up the tongue to touch the roof of the mouth and push hard for the seven second count. This is excellent for the muscles of the throat and chin and helps prevent the formation of wrinkles and sag in this part of the face. Press up the lower corners of your lips while resisting with the upper corners.

Curl up your toes, as if trying to hold a pencil. Do this fairly hard and contract the calf muscle at the same moment. Finally cross your ankles, left over right, and push them together as hard as you can, contracting the muscles at the same time. Change over and repeat.

With a little practice *all* these movements can be carried out easily. That's all there is to it. You can see why I call them my 'no time at all' movements. You cannot fall back on the 'I'm too busy . . .' or 'I'm too tired . . .' excuse any longer. It must be the easiest way in the world of keeping your muscles in shape. Remember – don't just stand there: Exercise!

Walk your way to fitness

So far I have described specific massages and exercises that need to be performed in addition to everyday activities. The final Body Sense technique I want to talk about should become a normal part of your daily routine, something which comes as naturally as breathing.

Next time you are on a busy city street, pause for a moment and watch the way people move around. In the space of five minutes you are likely to witness at least a dozen examples of individuals walking their way straight into the doctor's consulting room or onto the osteopath's couch.

It is not *what* they are doing which is so harmful to their health but *how*. Notice their posture. See how many backs are hunched, how many shoulders are allowed to sag, how many stomachs droop. Observe the way feet frequently trail along the pavements or waddle from side to side with every step. You may also get the chance to watch somebody moving naturally, gracefully and effortlessly with a correct posture and easy stride. It is not difficult to spot people like this because they stand out from the shuffling throng almost as if a spotlight were turned on them.

Movement and posture are vital but usually neglected aspects of health care. Fitness is not just a question of feeling good when more or less stationary, but of knowing how to carry bodily harmony into every activity you undertake.

Let me take the example of back posture because this is the cause of so much pain and so many problems. To illustrate how correct body movements help to prevent such difficulties, you need only hold a matchstick completely upright and try to snap it. In a vertical position, with all the weight pressing down from the top, even a match has considerable strength. But incline that same match only a little and it will break with ease.

The same things happen with the bones of the spinal column. When all your weight is directed downwards, as nature intended, the spine is as strong as any other bone in the body, and more robust than many. Curve the spine, even slightly, apply the same degree of stress and you are asking the vertebrae to perform a task for which they were never intended. They are unlikely to break but may well slip out of place. Such a displacement, a slipped disc when extreme, often causes considerable pain as so many nerve tracks run up the backbone. Good posture not only lessens the likelihood of these unpleasant events, but also improves health in many unexpected ways – such as by inducing correct breathing by taking the strain off the heart and lungs.

Because of the way the nervous system works, however, poor posture need not be felt in the back itself but can lead to discomfort in areas of the body far removed from the source of the trouble. Pain signals travel not only along nerve fibres but also through the bloodstream via chemical messengers called hormones. Bad posture also leads to the crowding of internal organs which, as I have already mentioned, causes them to work less efficiently.

Think of your body as a complicated machine which is moved around by rods (bones) and springs (muscles and tendons). Because of its design, this machine can only operate with maximum efficiency over a fairly limited range of movements. Beyond this range it may still function, after a fashion, but the actions will be less efficient and wear and tear far greater. Too much strain may be placed on the rods while the springs will either be stretched too far or not sufficiently. When the system is used as nature intended the same investment or energy goes much further. Not only is wear kept to a minimum but you can do far more without fatigue. So endurance and stamina increase and the effective life of the body is prolonged. All we mean by good posture is that you allow the body to work according to its natural design needs.

What does such posture involve? Certainly not the rigid stance beloved of drill sergeants. The idea of standing bolt upright, shoulders drawn back, chest thrust out and chin angled towards the sky has nothing in common with the effortless, graceful type of movements I want you to develop.

Teach yourself perfect poise

Try to set aside fifteen minutes a day, at least three times a week, to carry out the exercises I am going to describe. It will be easier to learn the movements while observing yourself in a full length mirror. Once you are accustomed to a particular way of holding your body while standing still, start to do the same thing when moving around the room. Learn to use your greater awareness of sixth sense signals to alert you to any deviations from a natural posture. Listen to the body. It will tell you whether a particular activity is being carried out in a health enhancing or a muscle damaging manner. At first, deliberately check on the way your body is working. For instance while walking down the street, turn your mind inwards for a moment. Think about how you are holding your head and shoulders, notice the way you are walking. Try to locate even the slightest amount of needless tension in any part of the body. Pay special attention to those prime target areas of stress and strain: the neck and facial muscles. While you are sitting in a cinema or theatre, or at home watching TV, switch off from the programme and switch on the signals from your sixth sense. How are you holding yourself in the chair? Is there tension where none is needed? Are you holding your head awkwardly? Is your lower back well supported? When distracted it is very easy to impose tremendous strains on the body. Only when the distraction is over do you realise how stiff or painful some set of muscles have become.

Be especially alert if you are obliged to stay in one place any longer than about thirty minutes, while driving or flying for instance, when sitting behind a desk or working at a factory bench. Pause for a moment to get back in touch with yourself. Go around the muscle groups in turn and demand a situation report. You will not need to ask twice. Immediately that part of the body which has become the focus of your attention will respond with information about how it is feeling and whether you are unwittingly causing harm to its efficient functioning.

Now for the exercises. I shall start by giving you four posture improving techniques then go on to look at the correct way of carrying out everyday tasks so that you are working with the natural design of the body rather than fighting it.

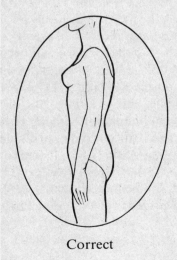

Correct

Fig. 122

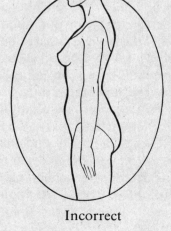

Incorrect

Fig. 123

Tuck in your tail so that the spine is straight as in Figure 122 and not curved as in Figure 123. You will find that this tends to pull in the stomach. Keep the buttock muscles taught. Improve matters further by drawing in the muscles even more to give yourself a flat abdomen. This one step alone will greatly reduce the chances of your developing lower back problems.

Lift your ribcage. This is done by lengthening the waist, just as you might open an accordion. Drop your shoulders down and keep them relaxed. They must not be allowed to droop forward, nor should they be rigidly pulled back, military fashion.

Keep your chin parallel to the floor. Pretend that you are a puppet with two strings, one attached to each ear, holding up your head. Now imagine that somebody is drawing these two strings upwards with an even pressure. Try to feel that your head is light and floats like a balloon. Learn to carry yourself with the head in this position. Do not tilt your head back. This not only looks strained but causes stiffness to the neck and shoulder muscles.

I must emphasise that when you are practising this posture there should be no feeling of stress anywhere in the body. Although you will be substantially increasing the tone in certain muscles, you should never allow yourself to become uncomfortable or unnaturally strained. A body moving in harmony with its own needs produces sensation of grace and a complete freedom from tension.

When somebody is moving correctly the focus of all bodily tension is the abdomen. This area is the body's natural centre of gravity and can act as a stable pivot around which the other parts are allowed to move. To enable it to carry out this task, nature has equipped the diaphragm with a broad sheath of muscle so making it capable of taking the strain from the other, longer muscles that control the limbs. The Japanese, who consider it to be the centre of the body's power, often wear special clothes, such as trousers baggy around the waist, designed to allow the *hara* – or stomach – abdomen to function optimally. Professional dancers move from their 'centre' to allow the rest of the body to remain relaxed and fluent.

Now let me offer some suggestions for ways of extending posture control into everyday situations.

When carrying heavy loads
The way you carry things like full shopping baskets, laden

briefcases or heavy suitcases, exerts a considerable influence on posture and muscle health. Most people realise the risks of straining themselves but still apply more brute force than commonsense to the task. When carrying anything the least bit heavy follow these simple rules to safeguard your muscles. Never use one hand only. The imbalance can easily pull your spine out of alignment. Nor is it any help to transport a single, heavy load first in one hand then the other. You do not balance out the strain in this way as some believe. The correct method is to divide all loads into two lighter ones. If you travel frequently use a pair of cases instead of a single large one. When you go shopping take two baskets, even if you only half fill both of them. On days when you know it will be necessary to bring back a load of papers or books from work take two containers. If it is impossible to avoid carrying a single, heavy load then the safest method is to hold it close to the body.

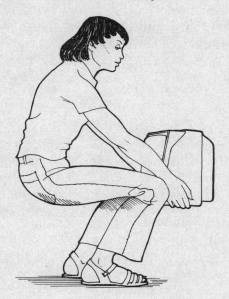

Fig. 124

When lifting heavy weights

Lift heavy weights as shown in the Figure 124. Picking up a heavy load incorrectly can lead to short-term discomfort and long term back problems. Remember that the spine is strongest when vertical so avoid any movements which bend it out of true. Come down to the object by bending your knees, and lift by straightening them again, keeping the spine upright and holding the load as close to your body as possible.

When sitting

The next time you are in company look at the different ways people sit and you will be able to make a shrewd guess which ones are likely to end up with back problems. Many of the positions adopted are unnatural and put a quite needless strain on the spine. When seated in a chair ensure the lower back is fully supported, by placing a small cushion between the lumbar area and the back of the chair if necessary.

When walking around

Keep your weight slightly forward and use a flowing stride, swinging your legs from the hips. Try to imagine you are being pushed forward by a gentle pressure against your behind. The average person lifts their knees too high and pulls, rather than pushes, themselves along. This increases fatigue because the body's natural forward motion is being inhibited. Move from the 'centre' of your system, that is from the stomach area, or 'hara.'

When in the office

Never remain seated in one position for too long. Move around regularly and carry out some of the quick exercises suggested earlier in this part of the book. In particular, move your shoulders and neck muscles. Change your copy from one side of the machine to the other every so often when typing. Try to ensure your working surfaces are at a height where you can work without bending forward.

When standing for long periods

Place one foot on a low stool or brick, changing legs periodically. Tuck seat under. Pull tummy in.

When lying in bed

Considering the amount of time we spend in bed – almost half our lives in some cases – it is astonishing how little thought is usually given to the way we sleep. Many people adopt such unnatural sleeping positions that it is not surprising their body feels far from rested when it is time to get up. Your choice of bed is the first consideration. Always sleep on one which is firm and provides good support for the body. Use only a small neck pillow and try to avoid sleeping face down since this places too much strain on the neck and lower back.

Back saver

Remember while driving your car to sit close enough to the wheel so that your legs are not completely extended on the pedals. Your lower back should be supported at all times.

Energy breathing

Don Ethan Miller, one of America's leading martial arts instructors, recommends 'energy breathing'. You can do this while sitting or standing. Breathe deeply and evenly through your nose, and exhale through your mouth, concentrating on your 'centre'. Now hold the breath for a few seconds just before you exhale. As you inhale imagine that you are drawing the life force of the Universe into your body, filling yourself with energy and sending it to every cell in your body. As you exhale imagine that your energy is extending outward to infinity to the very ends of the Universe. Between five and ten of these energy breath cycles will completely revitilise you. Try it and see!

The techniques which I have described will allow your natural powers of healing to make you look and feel in the best of health. Body Sense procedures can help you eliminate everyday discomforts, avoid unnecessary aches and pains, combat the effects of stress, enhance your appearance and enjoy a more active life.

When teaching my clients these methods, I have found that certain questions regularly crop up and, because a proper understanding of these key points is helpful in smoothing away early difficulties, I should like to outline these queries and my replies.

Q: *Which of the many techniques should I start with and how long should each session last?*
A: Choose the ones which are best suited to your current health needs. You may want to include procedures for relieving aches and pains or for preventing them in the future – the Awareness Analysis in Part Three will help to pinpoint any such potential difficulties.

After considering your current stress levels and looking at problems they may be causing, you might feel that a useful starting point would be to reduce the effects of stress. Alternatively, a more urgent task could be to work on aspects of your physical appearance which are currently making you feel negatively about yourself. If you are in good health at present then it may only be necessary to safeguard that sense of wellbeing by making use of the techniques described in Part Six.

So far as time is concerned, plan a schedule that allows you to use those exercises that seem most helpful. Make a realistic assessment of the time you can set aside each day for your Body Sense training and avoid being too ambitious at the start. It is much better to spend fifteen minutes daily, on a regular basis, than to confine yourself to an hour's practice every four or five days. Where possible I have given you the approximate times needed to complete each technique and this should allow you to create a reasonably accurate timetable.

I suggest that you keep a written note of the techniques to be carried out and work through them methodically so that you develop a routine which helps to sustain interest and to ensure that no key procedure is forgotten.

Q: *Can I use Body Sense techniques at any age?*
A: Absolutely. There is no age limit – upper or lower – at which Body Sense techniques do not make very good sense. As you grow older it becomes especially important to take extra time and trouble over your health and beauty needs. But if you are able to start at an early age, you can make life a lot easier for yourself in the future, both through setting up a regular routine of health care and by preventing needless discomforts and problems from arising in the first place. If you do begin when you are older, or if you are badly out of condition, then start slowly. Do not try to do too much too quickly or you may create rather than prevent problems. It is far better – and this applies to all age groups – to work your way slowly but surely into *any* new activity which makes physical demands on the body. Check out the situation with your doctor before undertaking any of our techniques if you are in the slightest doubt about your capacity to cope with the demands they will make.

Q: *Is the time of day important?*
A: Any time of day is fine for Body Sense training except after meals.

The Chinese, from whom some of the techniques I have described have been obtained, believe that early morning is the best time to carry out physical exercise. At day-break in any part of China you can see enthusiastic groups of men, women and children practising their exercises in public parks. Some people naturally feel more alive and alert early on in the day, while others only begin to get going in the afternoon or evening. You will know which period of the day produces the feelings of greatest energy and should take advantage of this natural response to help you feel good about taking care of your health.

Q: *Is it a good idea to carry out my training with a friend?*
A: Having a friend to work alongside you whenever possible is in some ways better than doing the exercises alone. While you do not actually need another person to help you carry out the specific techniques, their company will provide extra motivation to keep up a regular programme. You can encourage one another during periods when you feel more inclined to slip back into the old, less healthy approach to life, check on the way you are each carrying out the techniques and monitor one another's progress.

Q: *Can children use Body Sense techniques?*
A: They most certainly can – and should! I have seen children as young as eight or nine with the beginnings of postural problems, and they would certainly benefit from these techniques both immediately and in the future. For the healthy development of muscles, and an efficient circulation system, it is essential for children to acquire good posture very early in life. A surprising number of children also have problems with their weight, and Body Sense techniques can often help them back to a better physical and psychological shape.

Q: *How long before I will start to see results?*
A: It is hard to give a precise answer to this question because the time taken for a technique to work varies greatly from one individual to another. Pain relief should start to take effect after some 10–15 minutes, stress effects ought to diminish almost as soon as you put the techniques into effect. So far as the other benefits are concerned these will make themselves felt usually within a week or so of starting regular work with the Body Sense procedures. But do not become discouraged if it takes a bit longer than you expected. Keep working

and you will discover that perfect health need not be as elusive as you may now imagine.

Q: *When is the best time to start my Body Sense programme?*
A: As soon as you put down this book! It is only human nature to postpone any major change – and remember that Body Sense will be making a major difference to your lifestyle. To delay until you feel completely ready to begin, will probably mean that you are never going to start at all! Go ahead and start, even if you do not have every detail of each technique you want to use clearly sorted out in your mind. As you put my words into practice, you will anyhow become increasingly skilled in the use of Body Sense techniques. What is more, the great advantage of the methods I have described is that they are usually very effective even if not performed perfectly.

Q: *Should I take up jogging along with Body Sense methods?*
A: If you feel that is a way of exercising that appeals to you, then by all means do so. Here are a few tips that will enable you to get the most out of jogging.

When you first start jogging, take a rest between spells of vigorous activity. In other words, run a little then move slowly until your strength returns. Use your pulse as a guide to effective jogging, as follows. Subtract your age from 190, this gives you a peak pulse rate which should never be exceeded. For example somebody aged 40 would have a peak pulse rate of 150 beats per minute and the exercise should never be so vigorous or prolonged that the rate is faster than this. Monitor your pulse by feeling with your fingers along the line of the inner wrist, just beneath the ball of the thumb. Note the beats over fifteen seconds and then multiply by four to get a rate per minute.

Warm up before a jogging session in a slow and relaxed manner by doing a few side bends and toe touches. Shake your legs in turn, allowing the ankles to flop around in a relaxed manner to loosen the muscles of the thighs, calves and ankles.

Run on grass whenever possible to minimise the strain on your legs and wear proper running shoes which provide the right kind of support for your feet. As you come to the end of your job, walk briskly for a short while to allow the muscles to wind down. You should never fling yourself on the ground or go home and immediately lie down.

Q: *How would Body Sense fit in with my sporting activities?*
A: Very well indeed. Many of the pain relief techniques will prove especially helpful if you suffer from strains or tired muscles as a result of taking part in sports. Most people believe that they take part in sports to get fit, but really the opposite is true. You should get fit in order to play sports! Remember to use the Body Sense techniques to warm up, for example by performing the Jazz Dancers movements (see page 154) as a muscle warmer.

Q: *I have read that facial exercise can be harmful to the skin, so can I safely use Body Sense face movements?*
A: Yes, they are safe and the proof of this will be found no further away than your mirror. Just be sure when massaging the face not to stretch the skin. This can be avoided by tensing the muscles in the part of the face which is being massaged. The same applies to facial exercises. Make sure you do not wrinkle one part of the face while working on another part.

Q: *When massaging myself I find difficulty in applying the techniques smoothly, what can I do to make it easier?*
A: By practising these techniques you will quickly improve the smoothness with which the massage is performed. But do not worry if, at the start, the techniques are not carried out exactly as you would wish. As I have already explained you can still get good results if, in the early days, they are not being performed perfectly. To make your massage techniques more comfortable you can also do the following exercises designed to increase the suppleness of hand movements: clench your fist, then flick your fingers out so they are fully extended, then drum your fingers vigorously against your palms as if playing the castanets. This will strengthen and make supple your fingers so leading to a stronger, more effective massage.

Q: *Is there any way I can use my mind to help my body when carrying out these techniques?*
A: There certainly is, and I want to spend a little time talking about this side of the Body Sense approach to perfect health because the effects of the mind on the body are extremely potent. I have already mentioned some of the ways in which mental processes can be used to enhance bodily functioning. Now I want to describe a particularly effective but frequently overlooked aspect of health and beauty. I call it . . .

The hidden powers of fantasy

As a youngster did you ever imagine yourself to be beautiful, strong, desirable, and surrounded by many friends? The chances are you entertained all these fantasies at some time or another and, perhaps, still do. Unfortunately we are frequently told as children, and usually believe as adults, that daydreaming is a waste of time, a cause of failure, or a source of unrealistic expectations. Because of these assumptions you may have felt, and may still feel, rather guilty about daydreaming. Well, I want to tell you right now to forget all the negative things you have heard about fantasy and start using it to achieve success in the quest for total wellbeing.

I am going to ask you to imagine, in great detail, exactly the sort of person you most want to be. If you would like to lose weight you must vividly picture in your mind's eye a new, slimmer, more attractive you. If you suffer from aches and pains, I want you to see yourself confidently moving about with no trace of discomfort. If you are overstressed, I want you to conjure up a vision of yourself smoothly gliding through the challenges and problems you face daily.

Will this prove to be a waste of time, a mere escapist strategy that can produce no practical results? Not a bit of it! I have found that fantasy is a powerful tool when helping my clients to achieve health and an attractive appearance. What is more, my findings are supported by a large amount of scientific and medical research. For instance Richard Suinn, at Stanford University in California, has found that Olympic skiers can be substantially improved simply by picturing winning performances on the slopes in their mind's eye. Richard Atkinson, also of Stanford University, recently established that the use of mental imagery can *treble* a person's ability to learn a foreign language, while physicians in Britain and America have discovered that the proper use of fantasy can contribute to the curing of serious illness.

The nice thing about creative daydreaming is that it may be used any time you are by yourself. You need no preparation, no particular items of equipment, and no special training in order to turn on to these hidden powers of the mind. The difference between this scientifically proven technique and mere idle daydreaming, is that you control your fantasies rather than allowing your mind to wander aimlessly.

Wherever you happen to be, just go through a few moments of quick relaxation. Do this by thinking about the different parts of your body, starting at the hands and working around the arms, shoulders, face, trunk and legs to the feet. Notice any unnecessary tension in the muscles. As you become more expert in Sixth Sense training such tensions will be readily apparent. Now unwind those tensions and leave the muscles nice and relaxed. Once you have eliminated as much physical tension as possible, build an appropriate image in your mind.

For instance, if you are overweight, imagine the fat dripping from your body like wax from a hot candle. Then spend some time creating an image of the final result, the slimmer you that has emerged from this process. If you have a pain in your back, imagine that this ache is a glowing red area – a hot spot inside the body. Now picture cooling water trickling down your spine and attacking that hot spot, easing away the pain by reducing the area with its soothing flow. If you are under stress, imagine yourself confronting one of the problems and dealing with it in a highly efficient and masterful way, coming up with all the right answers and finding the most appropriate comments to make.

Gradually involve the other senses in this image. *Hear* the sounds that would be involved, fat spitting from the candle, the hiss as the cool water brings the hot spot under control, the complimentary remarks that follow your successful problem-solving effort. *Feel* that situation as graphically as you can . . . *smell* the event as powerfully as possible. Slowly but surely build an image that is as powerful as it would be if you were actually present in such a situation, experiencing it with the five senses and observing it very accurately and intently.

Devote a few moments to each part of the image, both the current situation and what life would be like after it had been changed for the better in the way you imagine. This can best be done last thing at night or first thing in the morning, but it can be carried out at any time when you have a spare minute or two. Between sessions you need not try to recall the images because although no longer uppermost in the mind they will still be working their powerful influence in the subconscious recesses of your being.

Although the process by which such fantasy sessions bring about positive changes is not understood, there is no question about their effectiveness. They will help to produce the consequences you so desire and make success in that area of life a far greater possibility than failure.

Now is the time to stop reading and start doing. Begin from today onwards to put into practice the techniques of Body Sense that can help to transform your future for the better. I want you to think of these procedures not just as a collection of exercises and massages but, rather, as a new way of living your life. A way of life in which the sixth sense you have now discovered is used to unlock the powers of mind and body which can produce that state of perfect wellbeing which is your natural birthright.